Intrathecal Drug Therapy for Spasticity and Pain

The printing of this book has been supported by an unrestricted educational grant from Medtronic, Inc.

Springer

New York
Berlin
Heidelberg
Barcelona
Budapest
Hong Kong
London
Milan
Paris
Santa Clara
Singapore
Tokyo

Intrathecal Drug Therapy for Spasticity and Pain

Practical Patient Management

Janet M. Gianino
Michelle M. York
Judith A. Paice

Rush-Presbyterian-St. Luke's Medical Center,
Neuroscience Institute, Neurosurgery Division,
Chicago, Illinois

Foreword by Richard D. Penn

With 88 Illustrations

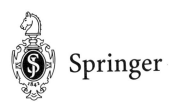 Springer

Janet M. Gianino, MS, RN
Rush - Presbyterian - St. Luke's
  Medical Center
Neurosurgery Division
1725 West Harrison Street
Chicago, IL 60612
USA

Michelle M. York, RN
Rush - Presbyterian - St. Luke's
  Medical Center
Neurosurgery Division
1725 West Harrison Street
Chicago, IL 60612
USA

Judith A. Paice, PhD, RN
Rush - Presbyterian - St. Luke's
  Medical Center
Neurosurgery Division
1725 West Harrison Street
Chicago, IL 60612
USA

Library of Congress Cataloging-in-Publication Data
Gianino, Janet M.
    Intrathecal drug therapy for spasticity and pain : practical
  patient management / by Janet M. Gianino, Michelle M. York, Judith
  A. Paice.
        p. cm.
    Includes bibliographical references.
    ISBN 0-387-94552-0 (hc : alk. paper)
    1. Antispasmodics. 2. Morphine. 3. Injections, Spinal.
  I. Title.
    [DNLM: 1. Muscle Spasticity — drug therapy. 2. Injections, Spinal.
  3. Pain — drug therapy. 4. Baclofen — therapeutic use. 5. Morphine —
  therapeutic use.   WE 550 G433i 1995]
  RM322.G52   1995
  615'.784 — dc20
                                                            95-19079

Printed on acid-free paper.

Production coordinated by Bill Imbornoni; manufacturing supervised by Jacqui Ashri.
Typeset by TechType Inc., Upper Saddle River, NJ.
Printed and bound by Maple-Vail, York, PA.
Printed in the United States of America.

9 8 7 6 5 4 3 2 1

ISBN 0-387-94552-0 Springer-Verlag New York Berlin Heidelberg

Foreword

The amazing thing about treating spasticity and pain by intrathecal drug infusion is how a minute amount of fluid containing a small amount of drug can have such a significant clinical effect. A typical intrathecal dose of medication is one hundred times less than the oral dose, yet produces a marked reduction in pain or the elimination of rigidity and spasms. To visualize how little fluid is infused, consider the average volume of 1/3 mL given per day by drug pump. A milliliter contains about 20 drops of fluid; therefore a single drop of fluid is infused every 3 to 4 hours. At this slow rate an observer would be unable to see the flow; it is so small that the fluid if in the air would evaporate before accumulating at the tip of the catheter. Infusing the medicine directly to the right area in the nervous system clearly makes a huge difference in how much is needed.

The tool for achieving this is equally amazing. The accuracy of the programmable implanted pump is higher than any other drug delivery system used in clinical medicine; it is better than ±5%, and it can go from a range of a small fraction of 1 mL to 2 mL per hour. Furthermore, the pump is reliable, giving what it is instructed to give and working in a continuous fashion for 3 to 5 years. As would be expected, the pump took many years to engineer and test, but it has been equal to the demands placed on it.

Properly using this new technology requires many skills. Though it is simple in concept, it is not necessarily so in application. Knowledge of the mechanics of the pump and the pharmacology of drug delivery, accuracy in the assessment of the patient's pain or spasticity, and correct diagnosis of complications are just a few of the requirements. The nurse practitioners who wrote this book have developed the necessary skills and, fortunately, taken the time from their busy schedules to write a guide to the successful management of this sometimes difficult but very rewarding new field of medicine. Beyond their technical skills and knowledge they have manifested kindness, concern, meticulousness, and dedication in working with our patients. Their willingness to share their expertise and experience to teach others the practical management skills they have developed is another example of their energy and generosity. They are models of what medical practitioners should strive to be in the challenging world of medicine.

RICHARD D. PENN, M.D.
Rush - Presbyterian - St. Luke's
Medical Center
Chicago, IL

Contents

Foreword by Richard D. Penn, MD v

1   Introduction.. 1

2   Spinal Cord Anatomy 3

3   Implantable Delivery Systems 15

4   The Operative Course 33

5   Pharmacology of Baclofen and Morphine 55

6   Intrathecal Baclofen for Spasticity 67
       Spasticity.. 67
       Current methods of treatment.............................. 76
       Benefits of reduced spasticity.............................. 80
       Patient selection.. 86
       Screening procedures 93
       Patient management 96
       Tolerance 118

7   Intraspinal Morphine for Pain 127
       Physiology of pain 128
       Intrathecal drug dosing 138
       Supplemental opioids.. 143
       Adverse intraspinal drug effects 146
       Patient education 149
       Case study.. 149

8   Mechanical System Complications 155

9   Starting Up a Program.. 173

10   Current Controversies and Future Applications 187

References   189

Appendixes

1   Baclofen Patient Teaching Booklet   201

2   Intrathecal Baclofen and Morphine: Policy and Procedure
(Rush-Presbyterian-St. Luke's Medical Center,
Chicago, IL)   207

3   Resources for Spasticity...   211

3.1   Patient Resources: Spasticity   211

3.2   Professional Resources: Spasticity   212

3.3   Patient Resources: Travel Assistance
for the Disabled..   212

4   Resources for Pain   213

4.1   Patient Resources: Pain...   213

4.2   Professional Resources: Pain......................................   214

5   Research Organizations   215

6   Electronic Support Groups...   217

1

Introduction

Centuries ago, natural products, such as plants, animals, or minerals, were ingested or applied to the skin to treat various disorders. For example, juices from the pods of the plant *Papaver somniferum*, a member of the poppy family, were used to relieve pain. It is only since the 1800s that chemically active compounds were synthesized from plants and other products into tablets, liquids, or topical solutions. Morphine, an essential agent used today in the treatment of pain, was first isolated in 1804 by Friedrich Wilhelm Sertürner. Since that time, pharmacologic advancements have led to the synthesis of many new agents to treat a variety of diseases and symptoms.

Methods of drug delivery have also advanced. Injectable compounds have been introduced, expanding the available methods of delivery, and the use of intravenous delivery has become popular in the past 50 years. Although oral, topical, and parenteral routes are useful, these delivery systems have significant limitations. Most of these routes deliver the drug widely throughout the body, leading to the desired effect, as well as possible side effects. As we learn more about the pharmacokinetics and pharmacodynamics of various agents, the specific site or sites of action are being identified. Thus, delivery to the site of action produces a more pronounced desired effect with fewer adverse effects.

Local delivery into the spinal cord is especially attractive in the treatment of spasticity and pain. Antispasmodic agents, such as baclofen, may produce significant central effects when given orally. The site of action of baclofen is within the spinal cord; thus delivery into this site would reduce spasticity at much lower doses when compared to oral administration, producing fewer central effects. Most patients in pain can tolerate oral opioids, yet a small percentage develop severe adverse effects to morphine. These patients might also benefit by delivery of drug into the spinal cord, a key anatomical site in pain processing, with fewer side effects.

The local delivery of drugs into the spinal cord began in 1901 in Japan with the intrathecal bolus injection of morphine by a physician named Kitagawa. The technology to chronically deliver intraspinal drugs progressed slowly until the 1960s. Indwelling reservoirs, such as the Ommaya reservoir, were introduced at that time to overcome barriers in chemotherapy administration to the brain.[1] External catheters, often attached to external pumps, were developed to improve intraspinal delivery. Technology has only recently allowed totally implanted systems to deliver drugs continuously into intraspinal spaces, minimizing complications such as infections.[2]

Although minimizing the risk associated with intraspinal delivery, the use of these more complex systems requires extensive training of health professionals caring for patients receiving this therapy. Knowledge is necessary of the mechanics of these systems, the pharmacokinetics of drugs intended for intraspinal delivery, and the specific needs of patients with neurologic disorders, cancer, and chronic nonmalignant pain who receive this therapy. The purpose of this book is to provide clinicians with the information necessary to provide safe and effective care to patients being treated with intraspinal agents for spasticity and pain. Where controversies exist in management, we have tried to present alternative views. Additionally, although every effort has been made to be thorough, no text can be completely comprehensive. Therefore, we have included other resources to assist in the care of these patients.

The use of intraspinal drug delivery has rapidly expanded with the advent of implantable systems. This expansion is likely to continue with the investigation of new compounds with larger structures, such as peptides and growth factors, for the treatment of spasticity, pain, other neuromuscular disorders, and even neurodegenerative diseases. Knowledgeable clinicians can make informed judgments while providing care for these patients as well as form collaborative relationships with basic investigators to advance the underlying science of this technique.

2

Spinal Cord Anatomy

The purpose of this chapter is to provide an overview of essential spine anatomy to assist the reader in understanding various structures of the central nervous system (CNS) and their relevance to intrathecal drug therapy. Structures such as the spine, spinal cord, meninges, cerebrospinal fluid, blood-brain barrier (BBB), blood supply, spinal roots, and spinal tracts will be addressed. Keeping current with this rapidly expanding body of knowledge directly affects the quality of patient care. It allows health care professionals to teach patients about the therapy, refines assessment skills, and provides safe and effective treatments that promote comfort and rehabilitation.

■ SPINE

The spine is a flexible column formed by a series of bones known as the vertebrae which provide support to the head and trunk. The vertebral column is made up of 33 vertebrae: 7 cervical, 12 thoracic, 5 lumbar, 5 sacral vertebrae fused into one structure, and 4 coccygeal vertebrae also fused into one structure. Each vertebra consists of two major parts — an anterior solid segment, or body, and a posterior segment, or arch. The cervical vertebrae are smaller than those in any other region of the spine. The thoracic vertebrae are intermediate in size, becoming larger as they descend in the vertebral column. These vertebrae may be easily identified by the presence of costal facets on the sides of the body and a transverse process which articulates with corresponding facets of the ribs. The lumbar vertebrae are the largest segments in the spine and are easily recognized by their size and by the absence of costal facets.

Health care professionals working with this therapy must be able to identify vertebral segments and their associated landmarks for many reasons. First, lumbar punctures, performed to introduce the screening dose of drug or to obtain samples of cerebrospinal fluid (CSF), require a needle puncture into the subarachnoid space between lumbar L_{3-4} or L_{4-5} segments. This location is a safe distance from the spinal cord, which ends at L_1. The landmark associated with this level is the superior aspect of the iliac crests. In addition, distinguishing between vertebral segments is useful when interpreting X-rays for catheter placement. Lastly, intrathecal catheters that are placed to facilitate continuous drug delivery are usually inserted at L_{3-4} or L_{4-5}. The tip of the catheter is guided upward in the subarachnoid space to rest at the desired site. For pain management, placement of the catheter may depend on the site of pain and is based on the physician's preference. When treating spasticity, the catheter is usually placed at the T_{12}-L_1 level. This level is considered ideal for catheter tip placement because it is adjacent to the neurons controlling motor neuron reflex excitability in the lower limbs. The T_{12} level may be approximately identified by locating the transverse processes that articulate with the costal facets.

■ SPINAL CORD

The spinal cord is roughly cylindrical in shape and occupies the upper two thirds of the vertebral canal. It begins at the foramen magnum at the base of the skull, where it is continuous with the medulla oblongata, and terminates inferiorly at the conus medullaris located at the caudal level of the first lumbar vertebra. Because the spinal cord is approximately 25 cm shorter than the vertebral columns, the lower segments of the spinal cord are not aligned opposite corresponding vertebrae. Thus, the lumbar and sacral spinal nerves have long roots, extending from their respective segments in the cord to the lumbar and sacral intervertebral foramina. These roots descend from the conus in a bundle known as the cauda equina. The nonneural filament referred to as the filum terminale continues caudally until it attaches to the second segment of the coccyx.

■ MENINGES

The spinal cord is surrounded by three meningeal sheaths which are continuous with those encapsulating the brain (Fig. 2.1). All three meninges surround the spinal nerve roots emerging from the spinal cord and are continuous with the connective tissue sheath of the peripheral nerves.

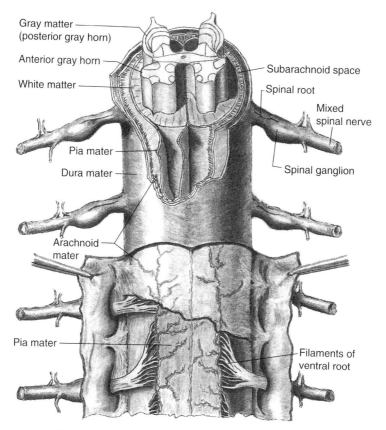

Figure 2.1. The spinal cord and its membranes.

The dura mater is the outermost fibrous membrane. It is dense and strong, surrounds the brain and spinal cord and merges with the filum terminale. The dural sheath lies loosely in the vertebral canal and is separated from the periosteum of the vertebral column by an epidural space. The epidural space may be referred to as a "potential space," and is composed of venous plexus and fatty tissue that may be used for drug delivery. The subdural space is capillary thin and surrounds the arachnoid membrane.

The nonvascular arachnoid membrane is the second meningeal layer that loosely encloses the brain and spine and merges with the filum terminale. This is the membrane that may become inflamed, a condition known as arachnoiditis. This thin, delicate membrane is separated from the pia mater by a wide subarachnoid space which is filled with CSF. This space is large enough to accommodate a small catheter, enabling medication delivery. The subarachnoid space is crossed by many fine strands of connective tissue, known as the arachnoid trabeculae, attributing to its spiderlike appearance. Blood vessels of various sizes are located in this space and may be damaged by lumbar or cisternal puncture, resulting in hemorrhage.[3]

The innermost layer of the meninges is called the pia mater. This highly vascular membrane closely invests the spinal cord. Because the diameter of the spinal cord is considerably smaller than the vertebral canal, the meninges and epidural fatty tissue fill the remaining space and serve to cushion the cord from the adjacent ligaments and bony processes of the vertebrae.[3]

It is important that health professionals be able to differentiate between the epidural and intrathecal space to understand the rate of drug absorption and the significance each route for drug delivery has on patient management (Table 2.1). The term "intraspinal" generally refers to all the potential spaces surrounding the cord into which medications can be delivered. Common use of this term may imply epidural or intrathecal spaces. The intrathecal space refers to the subarachnoid space, where CSF is located.

■ CEREBROSPINAL FLUID

The brain and spinal cord are suspended in CSF, a clear liquid that fills the ventricle of the brain and subarachnoid space. The average amount of fluid present in adults is estimated to be 100 to 150 mL (approximately 25 mL in the ventricles and 75 mL in the lumbar sac). Cerebrospinal fluid is constantly being produced by the choroid plexuses in the ventricles at an average rate of 0.37 mL/min, and the total volume is replaced several times daily.[5]

The CSF flows from the lateral ventricles through the foramina of Monro into the third ventricle, through the narrow cerebral aqueduct into the fourth ventricle, through the apertures of Luschka and Magendie. Cerebrospinal fluid slowly circulates in the subarachnoid spaces surrounding the brain and spinal cord. The bulk of the CSF enters the blood through narrow channels in the arachnoid villi, located between the subarachnoid space and superior sagittal sinus.

The CSF has many functions: (1) The CSF provides buoyancy for the brain, decreasing the weight of the brain on the skull, and serves as a mechanical cushion for the delicate brain and spinal cord protecting them from their adjacent bones. (2) The CSF removes waste products of

Table 2.1. Comparison of Intraspinal Routes for Delivery of Morphine and Baclofen.

	Epidural space	Intrathecal space
Characteristic composition	• Adipose tissue • Blood vessels • Connective tissue	• CSF
Rate of absorption (onset of action)	• Morphine: approximately 40 min • Baclofen: cannot administer into this space because the compound will not cross the meningeal membrane	• Morphine: approximately 20–30 min
Advantages for drug delivery	• Better for short-term morphine administration • No CSF leak • No spinal headache • Lower incidence of respiratory depression during a bolus • An early system infection does not necessarily proceed to a meningitis	• Better for long-term morphine administration because of a longer half-life • Less systemic effect because of less diffusion into fewer capillaries that are present • Fewer systemic side effects • Lower initial dose • Access to spinal fluid for sampling (cultures and drug levels), depending on the type of device used • No dural reaction around the catheter
Implications for nursing care	• Assess for risk of the catheter migrating into the intrathecal space and producing a potential overdose • Assess for untoward reactions, including nausea, vomiting, pruritus, and urinary retention	• Monitor for respiratory depression initially (morphine and baclofen) • Assess for a potential meningitis if a wound infection has occurred • Assess for CSF leaks and spinal headaches postoperatively

CSF = cerebrospinal fluid. (Reprinted with permission from Paice and Magolan.[4])

Table 2.2. Normal Spinal Fluid Findings.

Pressure (mm H_2O)	80–180 (when the patient is recumbent)
Appearance	Clear, colorless
Specific gravity	1.003–1.008
Cells/mm^3	0–10 (mainly lymphocytes; a cell count greater than 10 indicates disease)
Protein (mg/100 mL)	15–45
Glucose (mg/100mL)	40–60

metabolism, drugs, and other substances that diffuse into the brain from the blood. (3) The CSF plays an important role in integrating brain and peripheral endocrine functions; the hypothalamus secretes hormones or hormone-releasing factors into the extracellular space or directly into the CSF. (4) The CSF maintains a constant external environment for the cells of the nervous system, thus preserving homeostasis.[5]

The CSF has been regarded as an ultrafiltrate of blood plasma; however, CSF contains considerably less protein, glucose, and potassium than blood plasma. The CSF consists of water, protein, gases in solution (oxygen and carbon dioxide), sodium, potassium, chloride ions, glucose, and a few white blood cells, mostly lymphocytes (Table 2.2).

■ BLOOD-BRAIN BARRIER

The blood-brain barrier (BBB) is a mechanism by which large molecules in the blood are prevented from entering the parenchyma of the central nervous system through the capillaries. This barrier functions to maintain the internal stability of the CNS and, under normal physiologic conditions, often blocks medications from penetrating the brain and spinal cord. The BBB not only impedes transport, but can cause variability in drug delivery. The BBB is, however, permeable to water, glucose, oxygen, other gases, and lipid-soluble compounds such as morphine.

■ BLOOD SUPPLY

The spinal cord receives its blood supply from multiple radicular arteries which form the anterior and posterior spinal arteries. The radicular arteries arise from branches of neighboring arteries at the level of each vertebral segment. Radicular arteries enter the vertebral canal through the intravertebral foramen together with nerve roots. The anterior spinal artery extends down the entire length of the cord in the midline. Branches of this artery supply approximately the anterior two thirds of the spinal cord. The posterior spinal arteries are paired and extend inferiorly along the posterolateral aspect of the spinal cord. This artery distributes blood to the posterior third of the spinal cord. The outer aspect of the cord is supplied by small arteries from a plexus in the pia mater.[6]

The veins of the spinal cord drain into six tortuous longitudinal channels. These veins drain into many anterior and posterior radicular veins which empty into an epidural venous plexus. From the epidural venous plexus, blood is channeled into the external vertebral plexus, which eventually empties into the vertebral, intercostal, and lumbar veins.[6]

■ SPINAL ROOTS

The spinal cord receives and transmits impulses via nerve fibers in the spinal rootlets, roots, and spinal nerves and their branches. Nerve fibers emerge from the spinal cord in a paired, uninterrupted series of dorsal and ventral rootlets which join to form 31 pairs of nerve roots (8 cervical, 12 thoracic, 5 lumbar, 5 sacral, and 1 coccygeal). A dorsal and ventral nerve root join to form a spinal nerve which provides the innervation of a segment of the body.

The dorsal (sensory) roots consist of afferent fibers that transmit input from the sensory receptors in the body via the spinal nerves to the spinal cord. Cell bodies of these neurons are located in the dorsal root ganglia within the intravertebral foramina. There are two basic types of sensory fibers: The general somatic afferent (GSA) fibers carry sensory impulses for pain, temperature, touch, and proprioception from the skin, tendons, and joints[7] The general visceral afferent (GVA) fibers carry sensory impulses from the organs within the body.[7]

The ventral (motor) roots consist of efferent fibers that transmit output from the spinal cord. These fibers are classified as general somatic efferent (GSE) fibers which innervate voluntary striated muscles and general visceral efferent (GVE) fibers which influence the involuntary smooth muscles and glands.[8] These fibers are axons of (1) alpha motor neurons which transmit impulses to motor end plates of voluntary muscle fibers; (2) gamma motor neurons which transmit impulses to motor endings of intrafusal muscle cells of neuromuscular spindles; and (3) the preganglionic autonomic neurons which synapse with postganglionic neurons.[7] The alpha and gamma motor neurons are referred to as the lower motor neurons (LMNs). Each alpha motor neuron and the muscle fibers it innervates constitute a motor unit.[8]

Peripheral nerve fibers are classified by various criteria including their diameter, thickness of myelin, and speed of conduction. One classification system uses Roman numerals I–IV to subdivide nerve fibers based on their conduction velocity. Group I fibers are the quickest to conduct impulses. This group of fibers may be further subdivided into Ia fibers (primary sensory endings of the neuromuscular spindles) and Ib fibers (from Golgi tendon organs).[5] Group II afferent fibers originate in the spindle secondary afferents, which also come from muscle spindles.[5] In contrast, group III fibers are thinly myelinated, are activated by heat and mechanical stimuli, and are involved with fast pain of short duration and latency, described as sharp or pricking. Group IV fibers are unmyelinated, responsive to a variety of stimuli, and involved with slower pain of longer duration.[9]

Another commonly used classification system is designated by the capital letters A, B, and C to describe both sensory and motor fibers based on their thickness of myelin, diameter, and speed of conduction. Group A fibers are myelinated with a large diameter, ranging from 1 to 20 μm, and conduct impulses very rapidly.[7] This group of fibers may be further subdivided into alpha (α), beta (β), gamma (γ), and delta (δ). These fast fibers, specifically A(δ), are responsible for a short latency, stabbing, or pricking pain following tissue injury.[9] Group B fibers are also myelinated and exhibit rates of conduction that increase with an increase in fiber size. In contrast, group C fibers are unmyelinated with a small diameter, ranging from 0.5 to 1.5 μm and have the slowest conduction rate.[7] These fibers are responsive to a variety of stimuli and are responsible for the slower pain that follows a longer latency characterized as burning, aching, throbbing, poorly localized, and longer lasting.[9] Table 2.3 summarizes the classification of nerve fibers according to the two systems.

■ CROSS SECTION

The spinal cord is divided into the gray matter and the white matter. The gray matter consists of cell bodies, axons, dendrites, and glial cells.[8] Nerve fibers of the gray matter are oriented in the transverse plane. The gray matter is further subdivided into nuclei or laminae based on the microscopic appearance of the clustering of cell bodies of stained neurons by Rexed (1954)[10] (Fig. 2.2). Each lamina extends the entire length of the cord.

Table 2.3. Classification of Nerve Fibers.

Sensory and motor fibers	Sensory fibers	Largest fiber diameter	Fastest conduction velocity (m/sec)	General comments
A(α)	Ia	22	120	Motor: the large α motoneurons of lamina IX, innervating extrafusal muscle fibers Sensory: the primary afferents of muscle spindles
A(α)	Ib	22	120	Sensory: golgi tendon organs, touch and pressure receptors
A(β)	II	13	70	Motor: The motoneurons innervating both extrafusal and intrafusal (muscle spindle) muscle fibers
A(γ)		8		Sensory: The secondary afferents of muscle spindles, touch and pressure receptors, and pacinian corpuscles (vibratory sensors)
A(δ)	III	5	40	Motor: the small γ motoneurons of lamina IX, innervating intrafusal fibers (muscle spindles)
B		3	15	Sensory: small, lightly myelinated fibers; touch, pressure, pain, and temperature
			14	Motor: small, lightly myelinated preganglionic autonomic fibers
C	IV	1	2	Motor: all postganglionic autonomic fibers (all are unmyelinated) Sensory: unmyelinated pain and temperature fibers

(Reprinted with permission from Gilman and Newman.[5])

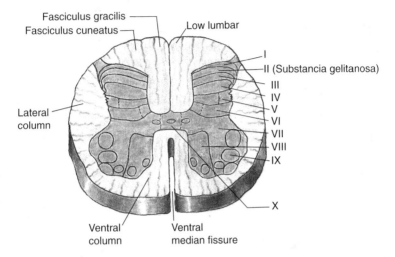

Figure 2.2. Lumbar cross section of the spinal cord illustrating the cytoarchitectural lamination, as first identified by Rexed (1952).[10]

Lamina I, the marginal zone, is an important sensory area for pain and temperature. Lamina II corresponds with the substantia gelatinosa, which receives information from nonmyelinated fibers and integrates this information with the thinly myelinated fibers that project to lamina I.[8] Lamina II is where the highest density of $GABA_B$ and opiate receptors are located.[11] Laminae III, IV, V, and VI correspond to the nucleus proprius, which integrates sensory input with information that descends from the brain.[12] Lamina VII contains Clarke's nucleus, which is present only in the thoracic and upper lumbar segments and which transmits impulses to the cerebellum about extremity position and movement.[12] Laminae VIII and IX are important for innervating skeletal muscle activity.[12] Lastly, lamina X surrounds the central canal and receives similar sensory input to that of laminae I and II.[12] The gray matter is also divided into a posterior horn (laminae I–IV), an intermediate zone (lamina VII), and an anterior horn (laminae VIII and IX).[8]

The white matter consists of myelinated and unmyelinated axons and glial cells that are oriented in a longitudinal plane parallel to the neuraxis.[8] The white matter comprises three bilaterally paired columns (funiculi): posterior, lateral, and anterior. Each funiculus contains ascending and descending tracts.

The spinal cord is enlarged at the cervical and lumbosacral levels to allow innervation of the upper and lower extremities. The cervical enlargement extends from C_4-T_1 segments with most of the corresponding spinal nerves forming the brachial plexus that supplies the upper extremities.[8] The lumbosacral enlargement extends from L_2-S_3 segments and with its corresponding nerves constitutes the lumbosacral plexus innervating the lower extremities.[8]

The spinal cord has intrinsic reflexes such as stretch reflexes and nociceptive withdrawal reflexes; however, its main function is to transmit impulses from the periphery to the brain and from the brain to the periphery. The tracts of the spinal cord are the structures that permit this communication with the brain. There are numerous sensory and motor tracts; however, only a few of the major tracts will be reviewed.

The major ascending (sensory) tracts are the lateral spinothalamic tract, posterior columns (fasciculus gracilis and cuneatus), and the ventral spinothalamic tract. The lateral spinothalamic tract is crossed, originates in the posterior horn, and conducts sensory impulses for pain and temperature. The fasciculus cuneatus is crossed, originates in the spinal cord at the thoracic and cervical levels, and transmits impulses for conscious proprioception and vibration from the upper body. The fasciculus gracilis is crossed, originates in spinal cord at the lumbar and sacral levels, and transmits impulses for conscious proprioception and vibration from the lower body. The anterior spinothalamic tract is crossed, originates in the posterior horn, and conducts sensory impulses for light touch and pressure from the trunk and extremities.[6]

The principal descending (motor) tracts are the lateral and anterior corticospinal tracts and the reticulospinal and vestibulospinal tracts. The lateral corticospinal tract, often referred to as the pyramidal tract, originates in the motor cortex and controls voluntary muscle activity. Eighty percent to 90% of the nerve fibers from this tract cross at the medulla. The anterior corticospinal tract also originates in the motor cortex, does not cross (but rather synapses with) cells in lamina VIII, and carries impulses for initiating voluntary muscle activity. The reticulospinal and vestibulospinal tracts originate in the basal ganglia and comprise the extrapyramidal system which facilitates or inhibits muscle activity. The reticulospinal tract is uncrossed and may facilitate or inhibit the activity of the α and γ motor neurons. The vestibulospinal tract receives afferent fibers from the inner ear and cerebellum, facilitates extensor muscle activity, and inhibits flexor muscle activity associated with maintaining balance.[6]

In addition to these major tracts, there are two other areas where axons are located. Lissauer's tract contains branches of small-diameter fibers significant for transmitting pain information. The fasciculus proprius, located along the margin of the gray matter and the white matter, contains axons transmitting proprioceptive information to different areas of the spinal cord.

■ CONCLUSION

It is important that members of the health care team working with patients receiving intrathecal drugs have an understanding of spinal cord anatomy. This information facilitates comprehensive teaching, improves neurological assessment, is required for diagnosing system complications, and promotes safe practice.

3

Implantable
Delivery Systems

Initial attempts to bypass the BBB and deliver medications directly to their site of action in the CNS included access by multiple ventricular injections. Unfortunately, repeated injections may damage the brain and increase the patient's risk for infection. Later attempts at accessing the CNS included the Ommaya reservoir, which was an improvement because it is implanted, but which eventually becomes fibrosed and was difficult for caregivers to access. As a result, implanted delivery systems were developed allowing for easier access and long-term regional therapy.[13] Early drug pumps developed in the 1970s were used for delivering heparin, insulin, and chemotherapy. The 1980s marked the decade that expanded drug pump application for treating neurologic disorders such as pain, spasticity, Alzheimer's disease, and brain tumors. The 1990s is the decade heralding new applications. Currently, there are two delivery systems commercially available for intrathecal drug delivery. The Infusaid pump, manufactured by Shiley, Infusaid, Inc, Norwood, Mass, was the first pump used for intrathecal morphine therapy. The SynchroMed pump, manufactured by Medtronic, Inc, Minneapolis, Minn, was later developed, but with programming capability. These two delivery systems will be discussed further (Table 3.1). Each pump manufacturer has booklets available to patients regarding the delivery system and its application (Fig. 3.1).

■ INFUSAID PUMP

The Infusaid constant-flow pump (model 400) is an implanted drug delivery system that is intended for long-term therapy in ambulatory patients. It delivers a continuous drug flow to specific sites via a radiopaque, silicone rubber catheter. The pump is powered by a self-

Table 3.1. Comparison of the Infusaid pump (model 400) and the SynchroMed pump (models 8611H and 8615)

Characteristics	Infusaid	SynchroMed
External properties:		
Material	Titanium	Titanium
Thickness	27.5 mm	28 mm
Diameter	87 mm	70 mm
Access port	Yes	Model 8615 only
Drug reservoir:		
Material	Titanium	Titanium
Capacity	50 mL	18 mL
Dead space	3.5 mL	2.4 mL
Power source	Two-phase charging fluid	Lithium thionyl-chloride battery
Flow rate	Fixed (1–6 mL/d)	0.096 mL/d to 0.9 mL/h
Programmability	No	Yes
Device longevity	Limited by puncture Life of septum (~2000)	3–5 years
FDA-approved drugs:		
Intrathecal morphine*	No	Yes
Epidural morphine*	Yes	Yes
Intrathecal baclofen*	No	Yes
Intraarterial FUdR*	Yes	Yes
Local Amikacin sulfate*	Yes	No
Intravenous doxorubicin	No	Yes

*Refer to text for exact applications.

contained permanent inexhaustible energy source (similar to the freon present in most air conditioners). The Infusaid model 400 pump is commercially approved for the following conditions:

1. Epidural administration of preservative-free morphine in patients with cancer suffering from severe chronic pain who are no longer responsive to conventional forms of analgesia.

2. Intraarterial infusion of FUdR in patients with metastatic disease to the liver.

This pump has also been used for administering intrathecal baclofen in Europe and intrathecal morphine for nonmalignant pain in the United

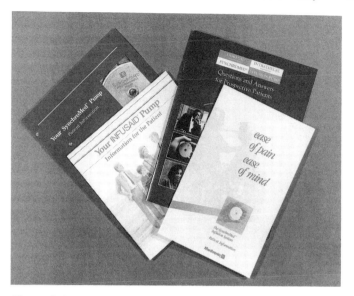

Figure 3.1. Manufacturer-specific patient-teaching booklets. (Courtesy of Medtronic, Inc, Minneapolis, Minn, and Pfizer Infusaid Inc, Norwood, Mass.)

States; however, these indications were allowed by investigative protocols.[14]

Infusaid manufactures two types of model 400 pumps. Each pump is a constant-flow pump. The single-catheter pump has a direct access port to the drug delivery catheter that bypasses the pump mechanism (Fig. 3.2). This access port allows bolus injections to be administered, which may supplement the continuous infusion and may be useful for objectively assessing catheter placement and regional perfusion by injecting radio-paque dyes. The model 400 dual-catheter pump is similar to the single-catheter pump except that it has a second sideport and silicone rubber catheter. The pump flow is divided equally between the two catheters, allowing drug delivery to more than one site. This pump is specifically designed and commercially approved for the local infusion of Amikacin sulfate in patients with osteomyelitis who have failed at least one course of systemic antibiotic therapy.[15]

The Infusaid implantable constant-flow pump is a titanium disk separated into two chambers by flexible metal bellows (Fig. 3.3). The centrally located silicone septum allows for percutaneous filling and emptying of the drug reservoir. The inner chamber is the 50-mL drug reservoir, and the outer chamber contains a two-phase charging fluid. The vapor pressure of the charging fluid exerts a constant pressure on the

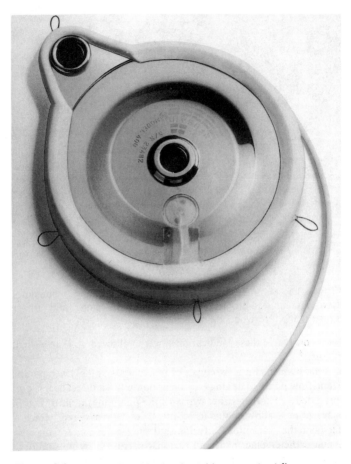

Figure 3.2. The Infusaid implantable constant-flow pump (model 400 single-catheter pump with side port). (Courtesy of Pfizer Infusaid Inc, Norwood, Mass.)

bellows, forcing drug from the reservoir through an outlet filter and fluid restrictor.[16] The drug then enters the catheter and is delivered to its site of action. When the pump is refilled, the increasing volume in the drug chamber exerts a pressure on the charging fluid, causing the vapor to condense to its liquid state.[15] The pump functions by maintaining a precise, preset drug flow for a specified amount of time. The amount of time depends on the flow rate set for that particular pump and the drug reservoir volume. Medication doses are changed by emptying the reser-

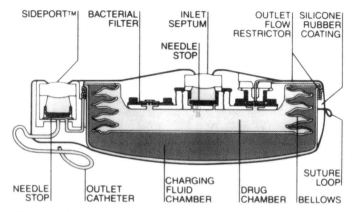

Figure 3.3. The Infusaid model 400 implantable pump (side view). (Courtesy of Pfizer Infusaid Inc, Norwood, Mass.)

voir of the remaining drug and refilling it with a new concentration of that drug. (See Fig. 3.4, a handy slide chart that calculates the drug concentration and refill interval.)

There are a few factors that may alter the preset flow rate of the pump for intrathecal or epidural drug delivery.

1. Any change in geographic attitude would affect the atmospheric pressure and consequently alter the pressure at the catheter discharge site. For example, changing from an attitude of sea level to an elevation of 6500 ft could increase the flow rate as much as 45%. This effect also occurs when traveling in commercial airplanes with pressurized cabins at 5000 ft.

2. A body temperature above 37°C will result in an increased pump flow rate of approximately 10% to 13% for each 1°C rise. In contrast, a decrease in temperature 1°C reduces drug flow by 10% to 13%.

3. The viscosity of the drug can influence flow rate.

4. The reservoir capacity can alter the flow rate because of altered pressure on the flexible bellows (at full volume, the flow rate will be 4% faster than the mean flow rate, and at lower volumes the flow rate will be approximately 4% slower).

Refill Procedure

Sterile technique is required for refilling this pump. It is recommended that the Infusaid refill kit be used to properly refill all Infusaid

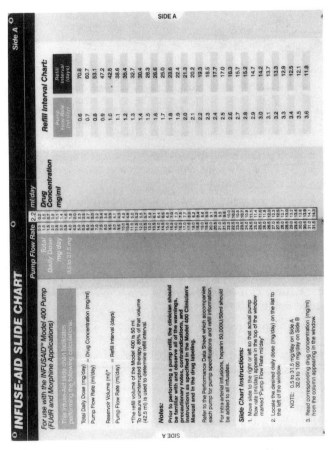

Figure 3.4. Handy slide chart useful for determining drug concentrations and the refill interval for patients receiving morphine and FUdR through the Infusaid model 400 pump. (Courtesy of Pfizer Infusaid Inc, Norwood, Mass.)

constant-flow pump models. Only 22-gauge Infusaid needles can be used to access the pump because other sizes or types of needles may impair septum integrity, potentially allowing drug to leak from the septum. After the outer perimeter of the pump is palpated, the skin is prepared using alcohol swab sticks, then iodine swab sticks, beginning at the center septum and working outward. A sterile template may be used to locate the center septum. Two syringes are attached to a stopcock and 22-gauge needle to perform the procedure.* Insert the needle into the septum of the pump at a perpendicular angle and allow the pump to empty completely. The pump must first be emptied of remaining medication. Note the amount of returned volume in the syringe and document the returned infusate. Inject 5 mL of the new medication into the pump. Release pressure on the plunger and allow a small amount of fluid to return into the syringe. This process confirms correct needle placement. Repeat this procedure in 5-mL increments until the syringe is emptied. Maintaining positive pressure on the plunger, clamp the tubing and gently pull the needle out of the center septum. Apply gentle pressure over the puncture site. Cleanse the skin of the iodine and apply an adhesive bandage.* Only preservative-free solutions may be delivered intraspinally (preservative-free normal saline, preservative-free morphine) because preservations may be toxic to the spinal cord structures (see Chapter 5).

To determine the refill interval, the following equation may be used:

$$\frac{\text{Pump reservoir}}{\text{volume (mL)}} \div \frac{\text{Pump flow rate}}{\text{(mL/day)}} = \frac{\text{Maximum refill interval}}{\text{(days)}}$$

It is recommended that the pump be refilled before it completely empties because the flow rate significantly decreases below 4 mL. This is important when accessing the drug reservoir; a passive backflow of remaining medication should accumulate in the syringe, confirming correct needle placement.

To determine drug concentration, the following equation may be used:

$$\frac{\text{Daily dose}}{\text{(mg/day)}} \div \frac{\text{Pump flow rate}}{\text{(mL/day)}} = \frac{\text{Drug concentration}}{\text{(mg/mL)}}$$

■ SYNCHROMED PUMP

Medtronic, Inc., manufactures the SynchroMed drug administration system. The SynchroMed pump is implantable, programmable, and indicated for site-specific delivery of medications for treatment of

---

*Refer to the Infusaid clinician's manual and the videotape entitled "Implantation Infusion Pump Refill Procedure" for specific instructions on performing this procedure.
*To access the sideport, refer to the specific instructions in the Clinician's Manual.

chronic diseases. This system includes a titanium pump, catheter, and external programmer which monitors and programs the pump (Fig. 3.5).

The pump is driven by an integral step motor which is controlled by pulses from a battery-powered source.[16] Battery longevity is a function of flow rate, lasting approximately 3 to 5 years. A collapsible 18-mL reservoir stores the drug. A miniature peristaltic pump removes drug from the reservoir through a bacteriostatic filter and meters it out to the catheter port. This pump allows a delivery accuracy of $\pm 15\%$ under a wide range of environmental conditions.[16]

The pump is equipped with two safety features, an alarm system, and a bacterial retentive filter. An audible alarm system in the pump sounds when the battery is low or when the reservoir volume is low. Using the alarm is optional; the alarms may be postponed or inactivated depending on the patient's prescription. A 0.22-μm bacterial retentive filter is built into the pump to filter the drug as it passes from the reservoir to the peristaltic pump and catheter port outlet. The filter is an important feature because it prohibits contaminants from entering the spinal cord and potentially leading to meningitis.

The SynchroMed pump model 8615s is designed with a screen apparatus located over the sideport that can only be accessed with a 25-gauge or smaller needle. This pump model was specifically designed to promote safety and prevent accidental refills into the side port, which lead to serious overdoses (Fig. 3.6).

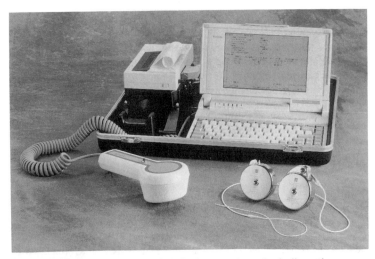

Figure 3.5. The SynchroMed infusion system including the pump models 8611H and 8615, spinal catheter, and portable programmer. (Courtesy of Medtronic, Inc, Minneapolis, Minn.)

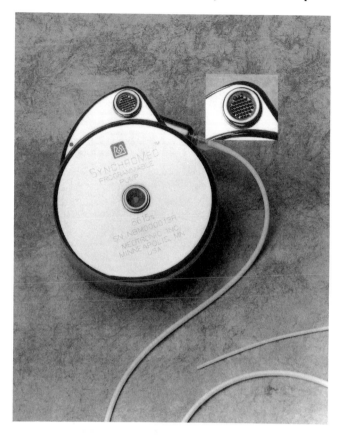

Figure 3.6. The SynchroMed pump model 8615s includes a screen over the side port which can only be accessed with a 25-gauge or smaller needle. This pump was designed to prevent inadvertent refills into the side port causing serious overdoses. (Courtesy of Medtronic, Inc, Minneapolis, Minn.)

An antenna permits communication with the external programmer via radio frequency telemetry (Fig. 3.7). The external programmer resembles a personal computer including a keyboard, screen, and printer. It also includes a programming wand with an antenna to communicate via a radio signal to the pump. The programming wand interrogates the pump and displays the current status onto the screen and printer. The user programs updated information about medication, concentration, volume, and dosage in common terminology that is telemetrically transmitted back to the pump.

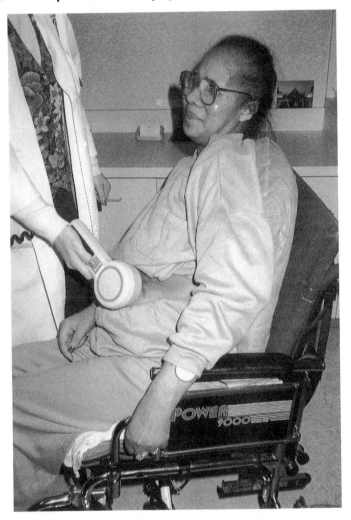

Figure 3.7. Communication with the SynchroMed pump is facilitated by a radiotelemetry link between the pump and external programming wand.

The programmability of the device allows flexible dosing options which may enhance therapeutic efficacy. Doses can be precisely titrated, noninvasively according to specific requirements of the individual or toxicity of the medication. Table 3.2 outlines all the possible delivery modes that can be programmed into the SynchroMed pump.

Table 3.2. Optional infusion modes.

Infusion mode	Graph	Description of delivery
Bolus		• Drug is dispensed once, usually at the maximum rate. • Prescribed dose can be set to infuse over a specified amount of time. • Used for trouble-shooting for system complications, supplementing a continuous infusion and when changing concentrations of drug.
Continuous cycle		• A constant amount of drug infuses at a specified hourly rate.
Contnuous-complex cycle		• Drug is administered continuously, but at varying rates at specified times. • A repeated series of 2–10 steps may be used. • Shown is a 2-step cycle; a 24-hour period is usually programmed.
Periodic bolus (bolus-delay) cycle		• Intermittent delivery of drug at specified intervals.

(Adapted with permission from Medtronic.[16])

The SynchroMed Infusion System is FDA approved for the following indications:

1. Chronic intravascular infusion of floxuridine or doxorubicin in addition to the nontherapeutic use of bacteriostatic water, physiological saline, and/or heparin when needed to support this mode of cancer therapy.

2. Regional intraarterial infusion of floxuridine used in managing unresectable solid colorectal tumors metastatic to the liver.

3. Systemic intravenous infusion of doxorubicin used in managing various solid tumors, lymphomas, and leukemias.

4. Intraspinal (epidural/intrathecal) infusion of preservative-free morphine sulfate in the treatment of chronic, intractable pain (models 8611H, 8615, and 8615s only).

5. Intrathecal infusion of baclofen for chronic, intractable spasticity of spinal origin (models 8611H, 8615, and 8615s only).

Refill Procedure

Sterile technique is required for refilling the pump. It is recommended that the appropriate refill kit be used to assure accurate refilling. The outer perimeter of the pump is palpated and the skin is prepped with iodine in a circular motion beginning at the center of the pump and working outward. A template provided in the refill kit is useful for locating the center septum. It is important to use this template when accessing a pump with a side port (model 8615) or separate access port because the possibility of accidently refilling in the side port could result in a serious overdose (Figure 3.8).

Assemble the Huber-type needle, extension tubing set, and empty 20-mL syringe. Access the pump reservoir by inserting the needle through the template center hole and into the pump's septum until the needle touches the needle stop. Withdraw the fluid from the reservoir using gentle negative pressure; air bubbles may be seen. Clamp the tubing and remove the 20-mL syringe. Attach the 0.2-μm filter to the syringe containing the prescribed medication (18 mL maximal volume). Attach the pressure monitor to the 0.2-μm filter and purge the air from the filter/pressure pathways. Attach the syringe, filter, and pressure monitor to the extension tubing, open the clamp and slowly inject the medication. Gently remove the needle with attached tubing and syringe set. Apply gentle pressure over the puncture site with alcohol wipes and cleanse the skin of the iodine.*

---

*Refer to the technical instructions provided in the refill kits and videotape entitled SynchroMed Infusion System Refill Procedure, 2nd Edition, regarding specific instructions and precautions with this procedure. The pump may be overpressurized when refilled incorrectly and possibly malfunction.

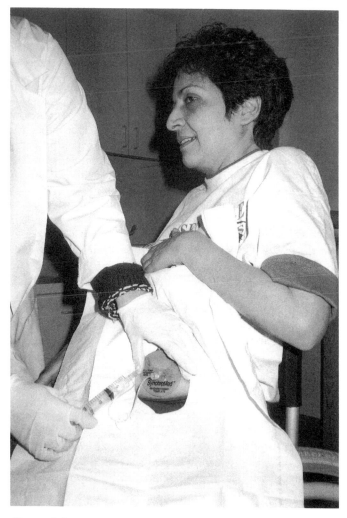

Figure 3.8. Refilling the SynchroMed pump using a template.

The refill interval may be calculated by the following equation:

$$\text{Refill interval} = \frac{\text{Drug concentration} \times \text{Usable reservoir volume*}}{\text{Daily dose}}$$

---

*At least 2 mL is usually left in the drug reservoir before the pump is refilled.

ie.,

$$\frac{2000 \ \mu g/mL \ \times \ 16 \ mL}{430 \ \mu g/d} = 74 \ \text{days or 10 weeks}$$

When drug concentrations or solutions are changed, the remaining old drug in the pump tubing must be accounted for to prevent overdosing or underdosing the patient. A patient can potentially be overdosed when changing from a higher to a lower concentration. The opposite is true when changing from a lower concentration to a higher one; patients may experience a temporary increase in pain or spasticity until the new, higher concentration flows through the pump tubing and spinal catheter. High drug concentrations are recommended for patients electing to lengthen their refill intervals, thus lowering the pump's flow rate; however, there is a minimal flow rate that must be considered to assure accuracy with drug delivery. Refer to the Lioresal Intrathecal Therapy Reference Guide for specific programming procedures on safely changing drug concentrations or solutions.[17]

Several factors must be considered when selecting either delivery system:

1. The specific applications/indications. Current information regarding specific drugs and applications may be obtained directly form the manufacturer.

2. Cost.

3. The device should not be implanted in the presence of an infection.

4. The patient's body size must be large enough to accept the pump bulk.

5. Frequency of air travel (Infusaid pump).

6. The patient already has an implanted programmable medical device. For example, there is a possibility of cross-talk between a pacemaker and a programmable drug pump causing prescriptions to be inadvertently changed (Medtronic pump).

Each of the pumps are commercially available for different uses (Table 3.1). Patients treated with "off-label" medications through delivery systems will be discussed further in Chapters 6 and 7. The term off-label implies that medications are being used in pumps for indications for which they are not FDA approved. Examples of two such situations are (1) hydromorphone (Dilaudid) administered intrathecally for patients with pain unresponsive to intrathecal morphine, or (2) intrathecal morphine administered for patients with spasticity who may be tolerant to intrathecal baclofen. It is the physician's prerogative to prescribe medication based on clinical relevance, experience, and careful judgment. Depending on the drug used and standards of practice set by each institution, it may be necessary to obtain permission from the institutional review board for treatment using off-label drugs through implanted delivery systems.

■ CONCLUSION

At present there are two different delivery systems available in the United States to provide long-term intrathecal drug therapy: the Infusaid constant-flow pump, and the Medtronic programmable pump (Table 3.3). The advantages of using an Infusaid pump include reduced expense and the fact that the system does not require expensive equipment to operate it. In our experience, refilling this pump requires much physical exertion (50 mL of drug through a filter and a 22-gauge Huber needle), and titrating drug doses require that the pump must first be emptied of the remaining drug and refilled with a new concentration. Also, the Infusaid pump is fairly large, requiring that patients have sufficient body mass to accommodate its placement. This pump may not be practical for patients with chronic illnesses who are cachectic or emaciated. The Medtronic pump is physically smaller, but costs 20% more than the Infusaid pump, and requires expensive equipment to program it. The programmability feature, with its various dosing modes, allows convenience with changing drug doses and more specific titration to patient's needs.

Table 3.3. Common Questions from Patients Regarding
Implantable Pumps.

---

1. Can a patient with an implantable pump (Infusaid or Medtronic) have an MRI?

Yes, patients with either pump can have an MRI performed; however, the effects of the MRI on the SynchroMed Pump are unknown. Patients that have a programmable Medtronic pump should have the pump programmed "off" and the reservoir emptied of the drug during the test because of the possibility for overdose or underinfusion.[18] Patients who have an Infusaid pump require no special preparation.

2. Can a patient with an implantable pump (Infusaid or Medtronic) have a CAT scan?

Yes, patients with either pump may have this scan performed; however, the pump may grossly distort the image directly around the pump. The Medtronic pump does not need to be emptied or turned off.

3. Can a patient with an implantable pump (Infusaid or Medtronic) receive radiation therapy?

Infusaid pump: Yes. However, the radiation must be directed away from the pump, the pump may need to be relocated to a different area of the body.
Medtronic pump: No. Radiation therapy may destroy the pump circuitry. Consult the pump manufacturer technical division.

4. In the event of death, does the pump (Infusaid or Medtronic) need to be explanted before the body is cremated?

Yes. Because of the high amounts of heat used during this procedure, a small explosion can result. It is recommended that the pump be explanted before cremation is performed.

5.   Do patients need to be aware of significant pressure changes affecting flow rates in the Medtronic pump?

Extreme pressure changes such as those occurring from scuba diving and hyperbaric chamber therapy can cause the pump to temporarily underinfuse or overinfuse. The cabin pressure in commercial aircraft does not affect the pump flow rate.

6. Will I set off alarms at airports?

Depending on the sensitivity of the devices used at airports, courthouses, and other public buildings, it is very possible that you may set off the alarm. Always carry your identification card.

(Continued)

Table 3.3. (*Continued*)

---

7. Can I continue to engage in physical activity?

Yes. In fact, walking, swimming, gardening, golfing, tennis, and other physical activities can help keep you fit, will help improve your mood, and can serve as a distraction from the pain. You can participate in these exercises and others within several weeks after pump implantation. Check with your doctor or nurse to determine when you can resume your normal activities. Although the pumps are very sturdy, we do recommend that you avoid strenuous contact sports or other activities that might result in a blow to the pump, causing damage or pain.

8. Will this therapy cure my problem (cancer, back pain, multiple sclerosis, spinal cord injury, etc.)?

Intraspinal morphine is given to relieve pain. This will not cure a person's cancer, although these same pumps can be used to administer chemotherapy. Intraspinal morphine does not relieve the cause of back pain or other chronic pain problems. Intrathecal baclofen is given to reduce severe spasticity. It will not provide strength or cure disorders such as multiple sclerosis or spinal cord injuries.

9. Will everyone hear my alarm (Medtronic pump)?

We always schedule the next refill prior to the time the alarm will sound; however, if you are unable to return to the office in time, the low reservoir alarm will sound. Most people will not be able to hear the alarm. In fact, even you may not hear the alarm until you are in a quiet room. One patient described the sound like a pillow covering a wristwatch that beeps on the quarter hour.

10. Can I continue to use my microwave oven?

Yes, the microwaves that may emit from an oven do not affect the pump activity.

11. Will I hear radio signals from the pump?

Sorry, you will have to buy a radio. The pump does not pick up or send the type of signals used in radio or television.

4

The Operative
Course

The operative course, including pre-, intra-, and postoperative periods, is essential to the long-term success of intraspinal drug therapy. Because many patients and their caregivers are quite anxious about the surgical procedure, extensive education is necessary. Teaching related to the operative course will vary since some institutions will implement the screening (see Chapters 6 and 7) and operative procedure during the same hospital admission, whereas other institutions may do these procedures during separate hospital admissions. Also, to keep health care costs at a minimum, the surgical implant may be done on an outpatient basis; although this is not yet common owing to lack of monitoring at home and fears of a potential postoperative overdose. In any case, clinicians must be knowledgeable about the operative course to provide optimal care and to better educate patients.

■ PREOPERATIVE MANAGEMENT

Preoperative management incorporates patient teaching and care, including preoperative tests. Extensive teaching begins long before surgery in order for the patient to understand the rationale for intrathecal therapy and how the therapy will be of benefit. This teaching is then reinforced in the immediate preoperative period. Guidelines for patient teaching and care related to the operative phase are provided in this chapter and can be adapted to your institution or setting.

Reaffirm Benefits

Reaffirm benefits established during the screening phase along with the patient's commitment to intrathecal therapy. Patients may have an unrealistic expectation beyond what the therapy can provide. For example, patients receiving intrathecal morphine may expect absolute relief of pain, or patients receiving intrathecal baclofen who cannot ambulate may expect to regain this function. Benefits that patients attain may vary widely and typically include increased comfort, mobility, and possibly function. Some patients may attain only basic physiological improvements in physical care, sleep, bladder and bowel function, whereas others may resume advanced skills such as driving, going back to school, or returning to work. This increase in independence may enhance self-esteem and affect quality of life.

Along with discussion of benefits, the preoperative time may be used to reiterate the need for the patient's commitment and knowledge regarding the therapy. Patients should be aware of how often the pump needs to be refilled or, if mechanical problems occur, that a surgical intervention may be needed.

Discuss the Hospital Routine

Discussing the hospital routine may reduce anxiety, improve patient compliance, and help caregivers plan for special needs during the hospital stay. For example, patients with severe physical disabilities may need devices not available in the hospital, or some patients may feel more at ease bringing equipment from home. Include such issues as:

Routine preoperative tests (chemistry panel, hematology panel, chest X-ray, urinalysis, urine culture and sensitivity, and electrocardiogram (ECG) in adults)

Length of stay (typically 3 to 5 days)

Sleeping provisions for caregivers

Special accommodations (air mattress, hypoallergenic sheets, wheelchair space, etc.)

Hospital guidelines (i.e., visiting hours, smoking restrictions, etc.)

Hospital staff

Describe the Surgical Procedure

A written guide may be used with verbal teaching to enhance patient comprehension and to help decrease anxiety (see Appendix 1). Studies show that adults retain only 10% of the information given during a lecture. Retaining information may be even more difficult owing to anxiety or certain medications; therefore, written information and repetition are needed to retain information. The teaching method may vary, but the content should emphasize the following:

The Surgical Procedure:
  Operative time (typically 1.5 to 2 hours)
  Anesthesia (usually local with short acting intravenous sedatives or general)
  Devices (IV, apnea monitor or pulse oximetry, deep vein thrombosis (DVT) prevention)
  Preoperative tests (blood work, X-ray, urinalysis)

The Pump:
  Size of the pump (show model of pump)
  Pump may protrude slightly (easily covered with loose-fitting clothing)
  Location of pump placement (assess for optimal pump site)
  Size of the postoperative abdominal incision (typically 4 to 5 inches)
  Postoperative bruising around the pump (usually minimal)
  Frequency and rationale for pump replacement (approximately 3 to 5 years for programmable pump and indefinite for nonprogrammable pumps)
  Frequency of pump refill

The Catheter:
  Size of the catheter (show model of catheter)
  Size of lumbar incision (typically 1 to 2 inches)
  Postoperative bruising where the catheter was tunneled along the flank

The Postoperative Period:
  Postoperative pain (usually minimal)
  No dietary restrictions
  No activity restrictions
  Oral antispastic and pain medications tapered appropriately
  Effect of intrathecal therapy will be assessed by objective and subjective measures

Obtain Legal Consent

Obtain legal consent for the surgical procedure and for any investigational use of the drug and/or device. Employ policies and procedures instituted in your setting when obtaining legal consent.

Rule Out Infection

Infections must be ruled out and treated prior to surgery to prevent surgical complications, which may include meningitis. For example, infected pressure sores may increase the risk of deep pocket infections.[19]

A moderate urinary tract infection may not delay surgery; however, appropriate antibiotics should be given for that specific infection. Also, it is known that infections increase spasticity, which may interfere with baclofen's efficacy and create difficulty determining the optimal dose.

A simple preventive measure is an antibacterial scrub such as providone-iodine (Betadine) in the abdominal and lumbar region the night prior to surgery. More importantly, an antimicrobial prophylaxis is ordered on the day of surgery since a foreign device is being implanted.[20] The choice of antibiotics depends on physician preference and the type of infection. Typically, intravenous cefazolin (a first-generation cephalosporin) is used. Vancomycin may also be used in hospital settings where methicillin-resistant *Staphylococcus aureus* and *Staphylococcus epidermidis* are common or for patients allergic to penicillin or cephalosporin.[20] The prophylactic antibiotic is given in the 2-hour period prior to surgery and may be continued for a 24- to 48-hour period for optimal effectiveness.[21]

Discontinue Anticoagulant Therapy

Because of the immobility of many of these patients, anticoagulant therapy is frequently used. Anticoagulant therapy should be discontinued prior to the operative procedure to reduce the risk of an epidural hematoma. It is advisable to consult with the primary physician managing the anticoagulant therapy prior to tapering the drug. Anticoagulants are typically discontinued 3 to 7 days prior to surgery to obtain an optimal prothrombin time of at least 75% of normal. Platelet counts should also be obtained, especially for patients undergoing chemotherapy or with thrombocytopenia.[22]

Establish Routine Preoperative Orders

Establish routine preoperative orders according to your institution's policies and consult appropriate departments (anesthesia, neurology, neurosurgery, oncology, physical therapy, etc.) depending on the patient's history and needs. Routine orders in our institution include:

Lab work (chemistry profile, CBC with platelets, urinalysis, urine culture and sensitivity, PT/PTT, and clot to the blood bank)

Chest X-ray

ECG if appropriate for age and history

NPO after midnight

Antibiotic to be given prior to OR (tape to chart)

Intrathecal medication (tape to chart)

Programmer to OR (if programmable pump used)

Anesthesia to assess the patient

■ INTRAOPERATIVE MANAGEMENT

Intraoperative management is important to understand, even if the clinician caring for the patient is not directly involved with the operative procedure. Clinicians who understand the procedure will be able to provide the patient with a realistic view of what to expect in surgery.

Prior to beginning intrathecal therapy, the staff in the operating room needs to be knowledgeable about pump preparation and the actual procedure. The manufacturer of these devices can provide inservices and teaching tools (videos, posters, and manuals). Health care professionals must follow specific guidelines; however, some components of the operative procedure and pump preparation may vary.

Position

In surgery, the patient is placed in the lateral recumbent position (lateral decubitus) with the side where the pump will be implanted being upward. This gives access to both the lumbar and the abdominal region for catheter and pump placement (Fig. 4.1). It is also important to obtain access to both these regions if surgery is needed owing to a catheter problem that needs to be explored and/or repaired. If the pump is being replaced without catheter revision, the dorsal recumbent position (dorsal decubitus) is used.

Comfort and safety measures are essential in any position. Pillows or foam padding may be placed between the extremities. Lower extremities may be taped to limit involuntarily movement. In extreme cases, general anesthesia may be warranted in order to secure patients on the operating room table and provide maximum comfort.

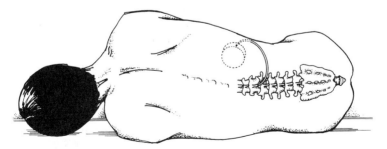

Figure 4.1. The lateral recumbent position allows access to both the lumbar and abdominal region for catheter and pump placement. (Courtesy of Medtronic, Inc, Minneapolis, Minn.)

Anesthesia

The anesthesia used during pump implantation is determined by many factors, including patients' history, age, physical impairments, and physician and patient preference. Anesthesia used for implantation of the intrathecal system includes epidural blocks, general blockade, general, and most commonly, conscious sedation with regional and local anesthetics. Conscious sedation is a technique used with intravenous (IV) drugs as supplements to regional and local anesthetics. The IV drugs used have a high clearance rate and a short elimination half-life. Patients receiving this technique are maintained with a minimal depressed level of consciousness with protective reflexes intact.[23] Typically, a drug combination of sedative-hypnotics and opioids is used. Sedative hypnotics may include propofol, midazolam, or diazepam. Opioids may include fentanyl, alfentanil, sufentanil, or even morphine. An antianxiety agent may be used preoperatively in some cases.

It may be necessary to give extra analgesics prior to the tunneling procedure, as this appears to cause the most pain and discomfort. Local anesthetics may also be used to reduce discomfort when tunnelling. Caution may be warranted when epidural morphine is used during the operative procedure and intrathecal baclofen is immediately initiated. In one case this resulted in hypotension and dyspnea.[24]

If the surgery includes only replacement of the pump, local anesthesia is commonly used, again depending on the patient's history. The patient usually spends an hour or 2 in outpatient recovery, then may be discharged.

Catheter Placement

The catheter is placed via lumbar puncture at vertebral level L_{3-4} or L_{4-5} using a Tuohy needle (Fig. 4.2). When the CSF flow is discernible (Fig. 4.3), a silastic catheter is threaded cephalad using a C-arm for verification of catheter placement (Fig. 4.4). Purse string sutures are placed at the puncture site to minimize CSF leakage (Fig. 4.5).

It is typical to advance the catheter tip to the lumbar or T_{12} region since this is an easily accessible area. At our institution, the catheter tip is advanced specifically at the L_1 vertebral region since the anatomical curve of the spine provides a more open area to distribute medication, which may possibly prevent catheter fibrosis. More importantly, because the lumbar-to-cisternal ratio is 4:1.1, central side effects are prevented since approximately only one fourth of the medication reaches the brain.[25] Since this drug concentration decline is gradual, a drug effect can be achieved in high thoracic or cervical regions by increasing the intrathecal dose substantially.[26]

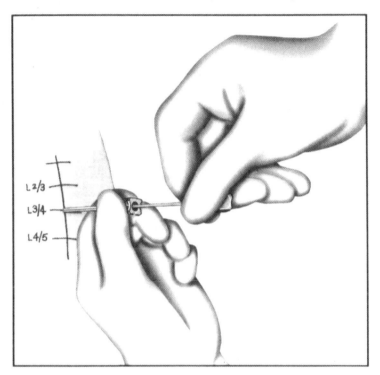

Figure 4.2. A Tuohy needle is percutaneously inserted into the intraspinal space at the L_3–L_4 level. (Courtesy of Medtronic, Inc, Minneapolis, Minn.)

However, a patient with spasticity in both lower and upper extremities presents a special problem. If the catheter tip is placed in the typical site between L_1 and T_{12} and the dose needs to be increased to be effective for the upper extremity, the lower extremity may be flaccid from this high dose. This may be a particular problem for ambulatory patients or patients who need the tone for transfers. Also, unless the patient is receiving anticoagulant therapy, flaccidity may lead to the development of deep vein thrombosis. The solution may be to place the catheter tip slightly higher, at the mid to upper thoracic regions. This should provide more even distribution of baclofen to sites within the spinal cord that control both upper and lower extremities.

For patients receiving intrathecal morphine for pain, the placement of the catheter tip may also vary. Some physicians prefer placement at the dermatomal level of pain (Fig. 4.6) whereas others prefer placement in the lumbar or T_{12} region, even in patients who have pain in the cervical region.[27]

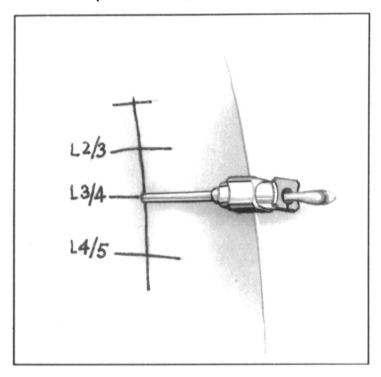

Figure 4.3. A backflow of CSF confirms placement of a Tuohy needle into the intrathecal space. (Courtesy of Medtronic, Inc. Minneapolis, Minn.)

After the catheter is placed in the desired location, CSF flow is once again confirmed by backflow (Fig. 4.7). The tunneling procedure is then performed using a passer shunt from the lumbar to the abdominal region, making a smooth curve with this instrument along the subcutaneous tissue. The force of pushing this instrument through the tissue may cause pain in patients receiving local sedation, and may also lead to ecchymosis.

Pump Preparation

In preparing a new pump it is *mandatory* to follow the manufacturer's guide carefully, as improper preparation could destroy the pump and possibly lead to overdose. Specific guidelines and teaching instructions are established by both manufacturers and include manuals, videotapes, posters, and assistance with troubleshooting. These guidelines must be followed and generally include the following:

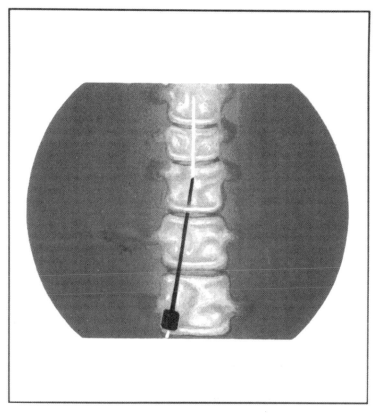

Figure 4.4. A silastic catheter is advanced through the Tuohy needle and is threaded cephalad using a C-arm to verify catheter placement. (Courtesy of Medtronic, Inc, Minneapolis, Minn.)

Keep the pump sterile, as it cannot be resterilized

Examine the Infusaid pump for appropriate drug and therapy usage, as they are preset and are not interchangeable

Compare the pump serial number against either the Infusaid Pump Performance Data Sheet or the Medtronic calibration number and document

Maintain the pump in a warm sterile container at the specified temperature

Refill with the proper medication and proper concentration

Use caution not to overfill the pump

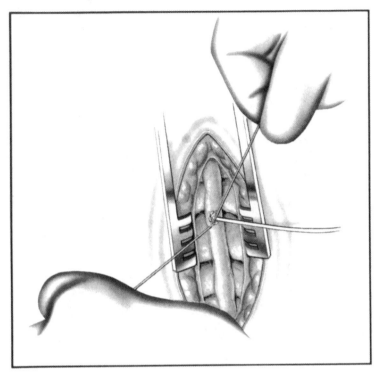

Figure 4.5. To minimize CSF leakage, purse string sutures are placed at the puncture site. (Courtesy of Medtronic, Inc, Minneapolis, Minn.)

Program appropriate information on programmable pumps

Prime the pump using guidelines from the manufacturer

Adhere to manufacturer guidelines for preparing the sideport

Pump Placement

The site where the pump will be implanted should be determined prior to surgery taking into account skin integrity, drainage, other devices or procedures that may hinder pump placement of a specific area, and patient preference. In rare cases where placement in the abdominal area is impossible, the pump has been placed in the subpectoral region under general anesthesia.[28]

Before the pump is inserted in the abdomen, the catheter is connected to the pump. The pump is then placed in the abdominal region about 2.5 cm, or 1 inch, below the skin surface. Caution should be taken not to implant the pump too deep, as access to the septum with a needle may be

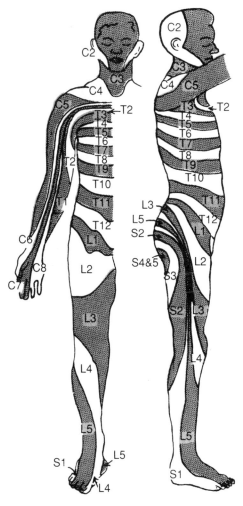

Figure 4.6. Each spinal nerve innervates a segmented portion of the skin referred to as a "dermatome." There are, however, no distinct borders between the adjacent dermatomes. For spasticity management with baclofen, most intrathecal catheter tips are placed at the T_{12}–L_1 level to produce the most dramatic effect. For managing pain with morphine, most intraspinal catheter tips rest in the lumbar region; however, some clinicians place catheter tips at higher levels within the spine, which represent the area of pain. (Reprinted with permission from Guyton[32] and Grinker and Saks. *Neurology.* Charles C. Thomas, Springfield, Ill: 1986.

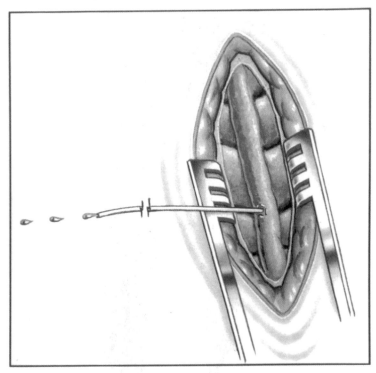

Figure 4.7. Once again, CSF is confirmed before the catheter is tunneled around the body and connected to the pump. (Courtesy of Medtronic, Inc, Minneapolis, Minn.)

difficult or impossible when refilling the pump. The extra catheter tubing is wrapped behind the pump. This reduces tension that may occur in the catheter during movement.

The pump is sutured into the underlying fascia in the pocket. Suturing the pump into the abdomen can be done either through the Dacron pouch (a thin mesh cover over the pump) or suture loops. Antibiotic solution is irrigated through the lumbar and abdominal regions prior to closing the wounds.

■ POSTOPERATIVE MANAGEMENT

Postoperative management includes a comprehensive pain and spasticity assessment, dose adjustments, and discharge instructions. Many patients recover quickly, returning back to their routine by the end of 1 week. On the other hand, recovery may take longer for some patients, especially those with debilitating conditions such as multiple sclerosis or cancer. A policy and procedure guideline may be needed for staff nurses who will be taking care of the patients during hospitalization. Refer to Appendix 2 for an example.

Routine Postoperative Care

Routine postoperative care is basic and should include the following:

Monitor respiratory status using apnea monitor or pulse oximeter

Resume diet as soon as tolerated

Encourage activity

Assess abdominal and lumbar incision every shift

Assess need for pain medication due to incisional pain (patients on previous opioids may require higher doses owing to tolerance)

Assess for changes in mentation or respiration every shift (twice a shift during the first 24 hours)

Continue antibiotic therapy for 24 to 48 hours as ordered

Dose Adjustments

Dose adjustments are typically done once or twice a day. Refer to Chapters 6 and 7 for specific information regarding dose adjustments for patients with spasticity and pain.

Discharge Instructions

Discharge instructions are helpful when given in written format and should be provided at a time that supports retention of the information. Refer to Table 4.1 for an example of written discharge instructions developed for patients receiving intrathecal baclofen. Discharge instructions should include the following:

First visit

Verify where visits are to be made

Remove sutures, typically 10 days after surgery

Calculate when pump needs to be refilled

Confirm next refill appointment

Infection awareness

Assess incisions daily for signs of infection

Call appropriate person if temperature > 101°F, headache, neck stiffness, nausea, drainage, or fluid accumulation

Table 4.1. Discharge Instructions: Intrathecal Baclofen.

Please return to see the nurse or doctor on _____

We will evaluate your spasticity, refill the pump with baclofen, and adjust your dose. The pump will be checked for accurate functioning.

Follow-up appointments last approximately 30 to 45 minutes and are scheduled every 4 to 12 weeks depending on the amount of baclofen you are receiving.

Medications: _____   _____
                _____   _____
                _____   _____

Never stop taking your oral antispastic medication abrubtly. Abrupt withdrawal of these medications can be very dangerous. We will give you a schedule to discontinue these medications gradually.

Activity:
Until your incisions have completely healed, avoid activities requiring excessive bending at the waist. Frequent transfers and heavy lifting may cause stress on the incisions.

After your incisions have healed you may resume your regular activities as tolerated (work, school, recreation, sexual activities, hobbies).

Wound care:
Check your incisions daily for redness, swelling, and drainage. If any of these symptoms appear or you experience persistent incisional pain, take your temperature and call your doctor or nurse immediately.

You may remove your bandage 2 to 3 days after surgery, at which time you may leave the incision uncovered and open to the air.

Do not take a tub bath until your stitches have been removed and the incisions have completely healed. Showering is permitted as long as you keep the incisions dry by covering them with gauze and a plastic wrap.

Sponge batheing is recommended.

Avoid wearing tight clothing, such as elastic waistbands and belts, that may irritate the incision.

Adverse effects:
Notify your doctor or nurse of the following adverse effects:

drowsiness   hypotonia
lightheadedness   nausea
slurred speech   itching
double or blurred vision

(Continued)

Table 4.1. (*Continued*)

Emergency instructions:

You will receive a Pump Implantation Card when you are discharged from the hospital. Carry this card with you at all times in case of an emergency.

In an emergency situation, such as extreme drowsiness or an abrupt onset of spasticity, call _____ .

Extreme drowsiness may be the result of an overdose and require immediate medical attention which may include a significant decrease in dose, monitoring heart and respiratory function, checking the system's performance, and possibly removing the drug from the pump or reversing the symptoms with intravenous medications.

Miscellaneous:

Inform family members and close friends of your baclofen pump, its purpose, and emergency instructions.

Remind your primary physician and dentist that you have an implanted pump prior to any medical or dental treatments.

Call your doctor or nurse if you should hear a beeping sound (alarm) coming from your pump. This alarm may indicate the baclofen reservoir is low or a low battery. If you plan to travel, notify your nurse in advance so a refill of baclofen can be arranged.

If you have any questions or concerns please feel free to contact us.

\# _____

\# _____

Reprinted with permission from Gianino J. Intrathecal baclofen for spinal spasticity: implications for nursing practice. *J Neurosci Nurs.* 1993; 25(4):254-264.

Wound care

Avoid activities that cause stress on the incision

Maintain dryness over incision site; change the dressings as necessary

Do not tub-bathe until sutures are removed; shower only if incision can be kept dry by occlusive dressing (a sponge bath is recommended)

Leave the incisions covered with clean gauze dressings for approximately 2 to 3 days after surgery, after which time the incisions may remain open to air

The gauze dressings may protect the fresh wounds from irritating clothing — for example, waistbands or abdominal binders

Medication
    Taper appropriate oral medications safely
    Continue analgesics for incisional pain as needed

Adverse effects
    Provide the name and phone number of a contact person for the
        patient to report any unusual side effects (headache, pruritus,
        drowsiness, dizziness, bowel or bladder problems, etc.)

Pump care
    What to do in emergency, whom to call, where to go
    Pump identification card (this is especially important if the patient
        plans to travel or enter buildings that screen for metal, such as
        airports or courthouses)
    What to do if the alarm goes off (if pump is programmable)
    Notify primary physician and dentist so prophylactic antibiotics can be
        given if dental or surgical procedures are planned
    Inform patient and physicians if special precautions need to be taken
        with tests or devices may that may interfere with the pump, such as
        MR or lithotripsy

■ POSTOPERATIVE COMPLICATIONS

Postoperative complications are rare, but it is important for the clinician,
patient, and caregiver to be aware of potential signs that may indicate the
onset of a complication. Signs and symptoms should be addressed during
discharge teaching; also, the patient and/or caregiver should be able to
contact the appropriate staff at any time since complications may not
occur until after the patient is discharged.

   Not all complications are severe. Fluid collection and spinal headaches
typically resolve without treatment. Although uncommon, infection and
severe spinal fluid leakage need immediate attention. Even more unusual
is an epidural hematoma which may lead to spinal cord compression
and requires emergency treatment. Although not a postoperative
complication, there has been report of a spinal cord compression which
occurred from an inflammatory tissue mass surrounding an intrathecal
catheter.[29]

   Adverse drug effects (see Chapters 6 and 7) and mechanical complications (Chapter 8) can also occur. Table 4.2 addresses postoperative
complications and their management.[22,30]

Table 4.2. Postoperative Complications.

Complication	Symptoms	Management
A. Spinal headache		
Because of CSF leakage during surgery, either to confirm catheter placement or owing to catheter penetration, there is always the possibility of a spinal headache (painful headache when either sitting or standing). The headache can last up to 10 days, or longer in severe cases.	Severe headache either when sitting or standing. Headache can last up to 10 days, or longer in severe cases (can be differentiated from headache due to meningitis, because meningitis may cause photophobia, nuchal rigidity, or spiking temperature, and the headache associated with meningitis rarely changes with position).	Having the patient stay in a recumbent position. Encouraging fluid intake. Providing medication such as Fiorinal to treat headache. In extreme cases, a blood patch may be necessary (injection of patient's own blood to seal the epidural puncture, usually done under fluoroscopy).
B. Fluid collection		
1. Serosanguineous fluid accumulation (seroma) may be noted the first few weeks.	Swelling over pump site. May be difficult to diagnose, especially in obese or larger-bodied patients.	Seromas typically resolve without intervention. If not diminished in approximately 2 weeks, the patient may be encouraged to wear an abdominal binder to decrease the pressure the fluid may be causing on the incision. If necessary, aspiration of the fluid using sterile technique may be warranted. *(Continued)*

Table 4.2. (Continued)

Complication	Symptoms	Management
2. Spinal hygromas (accumulation of CSF) are typically noted in the lumbar region.	Small localized area of swelling usually located over the lumbar incision site.	Also tend to resolve without intervention. If aspiration is required, there is a potential for meningitis. Because meningitis may occur if organisms are introduced into the CSF, aspiration must be conducted by the physician using strict aseptic technique. Surgical repair may be necessary.
3. CSF leak	May be noted by clear drainage from the wound in the lumbar region,* lumbar and/or abdominal swelling (CSF migrating through canal caused by catheter implantation) or complaints of spinal headache (see Spinal headache). A quick way to differentiate between CSF fluid and serosanguineous is to use the protein scale on the urine test strip.	CSF leak may require surgical intervention depending on the severity of symptoms (also see Spinal headache).
4. Epidural hematoma	Spinal cord compression	Although rare, an epidural hematoma warrants emergency attention with surgical intervention.

Table 4.2. (Continued)

Complication	Symptoms	Management
C. Wound dehiscence		
Wound dehiscence is a greater risk in debilitated patients with malnourishment. Any open skin area requires immediate attention.	Any skin area that exposes the pump or catheter should be immediately taken care of to prevent the patient from developing meningitis.	Management includes surgically repositioning the pump in either the same or opposite side of the abdomen. Prophylactic antibiotic therapy is typically initiated.
D. Infection		
1. Wound infection	Signs and symptoms may include erythema, increased temperature, purulent drainage, and tenderness of site upon palpatation.	Follow routine infection control procedure for your institution. Obtain cultures (from wound, reservoir, and/or CSF) and use systemic antibiotic therapy if appropriate. Removal and/or relocation of the drug pump may be necessary.
2. Bacterial meningitis	Severe headache, elevated temperature (101°–104°F), severe neck pain on flexion (nuchal rigidity), stiff neck, general malaise, a decrease in level of consciousness (may begin with drowsiness and decreased attention span), and extreme light sensitivity (photophobia) may be evident. *Kernig's* and *Brudzinski's* signs are tests of meningeal irritation.	

(Continued)

Table 4.2. *(Continued)*

Complication	Symptoms	Management
D. Infection *(continued)*		
2. Bacterial meningitis *(continued)*	*Kernig's sign:* have patient in recumbent position, flex one of the patient's legs at the hip and knee, then straighten the knee. Observe for resistance or pain. Note that this may be difficult to attempt in patients with spasticity, since infection increases spasticity. *Brudzinski's sign:* have patient in recumbent position, place your hands behind the patient's head and flex the neck forward. Note resistance or pain. Also watch for flexion of the patient's hips and knees in reaction to your maneuver.	Obtain cultures from the medication in the pump and from the CSF. Treat with appropriate antibiotics. Consider temporarily removing the pump. (One case of staphylococcal meningitis was treated with intrathecal vancomycin by the same pump.[30,31]

*Serosanguineous fluid is rich in protein and a urine test strip reading of 500 mg/dL or more is typical, whereas CSF has minimal protein.

■ CONCLUSION

Patients may be ambivalent about having a drug pump implanted in their body that dispenses medication directly into the spine. Extensive education about the delivery system and its safety along with reviewing the benefits with each patient is essential. The surgical procedure for implanting a drug pump and intraspinal catheter is a safe and nondestructive procedure creating no further neurologic impairment to the patient. Also, it is a relatively simple surgical procedure.

Postoperatively, doses of the intraspinal medication are titrated while supplemental systemic pain medications may be decreased and oral medications gradually discontinued. Patients must be assessed postoperatively for complications such as CSF leaks, meningitis, wound infections, and seromas. Explicit verbal and written discharge instructions must be provided for each individual and their family/caregiver.

5

Pharmacology of Baclofen and Morphine

Understanding the pharmacology of drugs intended for intraspinal use assists the clinician in patient management. Pharmacokinetic factors such as lipid solubility, pH and pK_a, molecular weight, and affinity must also be considered when comparing agents to use for specific patient conditions. The potential adverse effects of preservatives and antioxidants on spinal cord tissue must be weighed when considering agents that contain these compounds for intraspinal delivery. Specific agents will be discussed, with emphasis on baclofen and morphine but also addressing new categories of drugs that might be given intraspinally to treat spasticity and pain.

■ PHARMACOKINETIC FACTORS

Agents injected intraspinally reach the site of action in the spinal cord either by passive diffusion, as with intrathecal use, or by epidural injection, where the drug must first cross the dura and arachnoid membranes and then diffuse into the cord to the site of action.[33] For opioids and baclofen, these sites are primarily in laminae I and II in the dorsal horn. When given epidurally, several less direct pathways exist for drug to reach the site of action. For example, drug may be taken up by the vasculature in the epidural space and enter into systemic circulation, with a small amount eventually reaching opioid receptors in the spinal cord and brain. Drug may also enter through dural root sleeves and arachnoid villi, particularly during coughing or through the Valsalva maneuver. Drug may also be stored by the fat within the epidural space. From this fat depot, the drug can eventually enter into the systemic circulation or cross the dura to enter the CSF.[34]

The direct delivery of drugs into the intrathecal space is more efficient and predictable, since less drug reaches vascular or fat depots.[35] Because of the anatomical differences between these spaces, pharmacokinetic factors must be considered when choosing a drug for epidural or intrathecal use, particularly the lipid solubility of the solution.

Lipid Solubility/pH/pK_a

Drugs given epidurally must cross the dura and subarachnoid membranes before eventually diffusing into the gray matter of the spinal cord. Lipophilic drugs (agents that are soluble in fat) can cross membranes more rapidly and efficiently and thus are more useful when given epidurally.[36,37] Fentanyl, a commonly used opioid that is approximately 100 times more potent than morphine, is an example of a more lipophilic drug. However, when given intrathecally, lipophilic drugs may cross the dura mater back into the epidural space and enter the systemic circulation through the blood vessels in this space. A recent study of blood levels after epidural or intravenous administration of fentanyl for postthoracotomy pain suggests that the analgesic effect of epidural delivery is largely due to systemic uptake of the drug.[38]

As a result of the propensity for lipid-soluble agents to enter the systemic circulation, more hydrophilic (water-soluble) drugs, such as morphine, have been shown to be more potent when administered intrathecally.[39] Concern is often expressed regarding the possible delayed rostral flow of intrathecallyadministered hydrophilic drugs, leading to late-onset respiratory depression.[35] Rostral flow does occur during continuous drug delivery; in fact, our experience with both morphine and baclofen indicates that approximately 25% of the drug reaches the cisterna magna.[26] However, continuous administration leads to a steady state, with little variation in drug levels near the respiratory centers in the pons. The risk of late-onset respiratory depression associated with hydrophilic drugs is greater with bolus delivery, where a larger volume is rapidly injected, leading to greater amounts of drug ascending to higher centers. Table 5.1 indicates the solubility of various agents used intraspinally.

In addition to the lipid solubility of a drug, pH and pK_a also affect the way drugs cross membranes. Drugs that have no charge (those that are less ionized or nonpolar) diffuse across lipid-containing membranes more easily than positively or negatively charged (ionized or polar) agents.[41] Consequently, the ability of a drug to be transported through tissues to the site of action is dependent upon both the pH and pK_a of the drug. The pK_a of a drug, determined by the Henderson-Hasselbalch equation, is the pH at which a specific drug is 50% ionized and 50% nonionized. Because

Table 5.1. Physicochemical Properties* of Agents Commonly Administered by Implanted Pumps.

Drug	Molecular weight	pH	pK_a[†]	Partition coefficient[‡]
Baclofen	214	5.7	3.74–9.53 (has 2 pK_as)	0.1
Morphine	285	4.78	8.9	0.7
Hydromorphone	322	3.5–5.5	8.1–9.5	1.28
Bupivacaine	288	5.9	8.1	27.5
Fentanyl	336	5.73	8.4	717.0
Sufentanil	386	3.5–6.0	8.0	2842.0

*Physicochemical properties such as molecular weight, pH, pK_a, and partition coefficient affect the distribution of drugs given intraspinally.

†The pK_a is the pH at which a drug is 50% ionized.

‡The partition coefficient is the relative solubility of a drug. It can be measured by adding a drug to a mixture of oil and octanol (or ethanol) and determining the drug concentrations in each layer after the oil and octanol separate. The partition coefficients listed in this table reflect the following ratio:

$$\text{Partition coefficient} = \frac{\text{Drug concentration appearing in octanol}}{\text{Drug concentration appearing in water}}$$

Values greater than 1 reflect more lipid-soluble substances; larger values indicate greater solubility in lipids.

(Reprinted with permission from Paice and Williams[40])

the pH of the CSF is 7.3 to 7.4, any drug with a pK_a outside of this range will be ionized at the nearly neutral pH of the CSF. For example, more basic drugs with a pK_a greater than 7.4 will be more ionized at the pH of the CSF. Most opioids have a pK_a between 8 to 9; the pK_a of bupivicaine is 8.1.[34] When comparing various opioids, more ionized compounds (such as morphine and hydromorphone) have a slower onset of action when given intrathecally, and a longer duration of action than less ionized compounds (including fentanyl).

Molecular Weight

Because of their large size, high-molecular-weight compounds are less able to cross the dural membranes.[33] Most of the agents in current clinical use have similar molecular weights (Table 5.1). This may become of greater concern, however, as new drugs, including large peptide compounds, are considered for intraspinal use in the treatment of various neurological syndromes.

Affinity

Several factors relate to drug affinity, including the ability of a drug to bind with its specific receptor, the strength of binding, and the time the drug occupies the receptor. For example, morphine has a high level of affinity for its specific receptor, so morphine has a longer duration of action when administered intraspinally than fentanyl, which seems to have a comparatively low level of affinity for its specific receptor. Baclofen also has a moderately high level of affinity for the $GABA_B$ receptor.

Preservatives

Other concerns when administering drugs intraspinally include the use of preservatives and antioxidants. Alcohol, phenol, formaldehyde, and sodium metabisulfite are toxic to the central nervous system,[42-46] and their intraspinal use should be avoided. Any agent in a multiple-dose vial should be considered to contain preservatives.

Morphine can be reconstituted from powder or tablets intended for hypodermic use and filtered, but some antigens may pass through the filter. Preservative-free morphine is currently available in 10 mg/mL and 25 mg/mL solutions (Infumorph; Elkins-Sinn or Wyeth). Another alternative is the use of morphine with low concentrations of chlorobutanol, a derivative of chloroform. Long-term use of this solution is believed to be safe.[47] Hydromorphone (Dilaudid-HP; Knoll Pharmaceutical Company) is available in 10 mg/mL concentrations and contains the antioxidants sodium citrate and citric acid, which are nontoxic and natural components of living organisms. Although the equianalgesic conversion from intraspinal morphine to hydromorphone is unknown, systemic administration of hydromorphone is approximately 5 to 7 times more potent than morphine, allowing smaller volumes to be delivered. A recent survey suggests that hydromorphone is frequently used without adverse effects.[48] Fentanyl and sufentanil, approximately 100 and 1000 times more potent than morphine, respectively, are also available in preservative-free solutions and are commonly used in postoperative analgesia. Finally, baclofen (Lioresal intrathecal) is available in a preservative- and antioxidant-free formulation.

■ PHARMACOLOGY OF SPECIFIC AGENTS

Many drugs have been administered via implanted drug pumps (Table 5.2), although at this time, baclofen and morphine are the only agents approved by the FDA for intraspinal use. Baclofen, an agent used orally

Table 5.2. Agents Given Intraspinally.

Opiate agonists	Mixed or partial agonists
Morphine[†]	Tramadol[†]
Hydromorphone[†]	Butorphanol
Meperidine[†]	Buprenorphine
Methadone	Pentazocine
Heroin	Nalbuphine
Fentanyl[†]	
Sufentanil[†]	Anesthetic agents
Alfentanil	Lidocaine[†]
Lofentanil	Bupivacaine[†]
DADL[†]	Etidocaine
Endorphin	Lignocaine
Dynorphin	Tetracaine[†]
Morphine-6-glucuronide	
Met-enkephalin	Others
	Clonidine[†]
	Octreotide[†]
	Baclofen[*†]
	Calcitonin
	Ketamine
	Midazolam

*Morphine and baclofen are the only agents currently approved for use in implanted pumps in the United States. The use of other medications constitutes off-label use of a drug.
†Agents that have been given via implanted pumps.
Numberous agents have been given into the epidural or intrathecal space. Unfortunately, adequate toxicity testing of many of these drugs has not been conducted.
(Reprinted with permission from Paice and Buck.[49])

for many years, is currently administered intrathecally for the treatment of severe spasticity that does not respond adequately to oral treatment. Opioids are the most common agents used to relieve severe pain, although morphine is also used for drug holidays when tolerance develops to baclofen. Local anesthetics are used for severe neuropathic pain, described by patients as tingling, burning, and electrical. In some centers, local anesthetics are used for the treatment of spasticity as an alternative to baclofen. Finally, new agents are currently being examined for their efficacy in relieving pain and spasticity.

Baclofen

Baclofen (Lioresal) is a muscle relaxant and antispastic agent that is structurally related to gamma-aminobutyric acid (GABA). Baclofen binds to the $GABA_B$ receptors located in laminae II (also referred to as the substantia gelatinosa) and III to block mono- and polysynaptic reflexes.[11,50]

When administered orally, little baclofen reaches the CSF, which is due in part to the hydrophilic nature of the drug (Fig. 5.1). Hydrophilic agents are less able to cross membranes than lipophilic substances. Only a small amount of baclofen is able to cross the blood-brain barrier and reach the site of action within the spinal cord. As a result, larger oral doses are required, leading to CNS side effects, including sedation and confusion. Intraspinal administration provides direct delivery to the spinal cord. Less baclofen is required, and very little drug reaches supraspinal centers when compared to oral administration.

Animal studies preceded the use of intrathecal baclofen in humans. Intrathecal baclofen administered to rats and monkeys produced antinociception (pain relief) and at higher doses, flaccidity.[52,53] Single doses of intrathecal baclofen given to rabbits inhibited polysynaptic reflexes beginning within 15 minutes after the injection and lasting for 5 hours or longer.[54] No evidence of tissue irritation or inflammation was noted in the spinal cords of rabbits or cats receiving intermittent or chronic infusions of intrathecal baclofen,[53,54,55] supporting the safety of intrathecal use.

Clinical trials of intrathecal baclofen began using single bolus injections to establish the efficacy and safety of this technique. Patients with severe spasticity related to multiple sclerosis and spinal cord injury

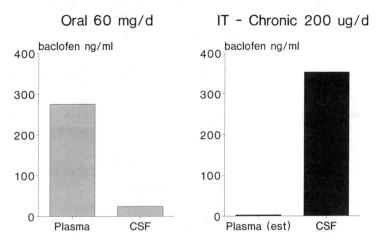

Figure 5.1. A comparison of plasma and CSF drug lends after oral and intrathecal baclofen administration. (Reprinted with permission from Penn R. and Kroin J. Intrathecal baclofen in the long-term management of severe spasticity. *Neurosurgery*. 1989; 4(2):325–332.

received a bolus dose of 25 to 100 μg, which produced normal muscle tone and the absence of spontaneous spasms.[25,56] No side effects were observed. The success of this trial led to the use of implanted pumps to deliver intrathecal baclofen.

The pharmacodynamics and pharmacokinetics of intrathecal baclofen have been established after use in large numbers of patients. Although wide variability exists between patients, the average time to respond to a continuous infusion of intrathecal baclofen is 6 to 8 hours after beginning the infusion, with maximum activity at 24 to 48 hours.[57] Bolus delivery of intrathecal baclofen usually relieves spasticity in approximately 1 hour.[56] The CSF clearance is generally 30 mL/hr, with approximately 25% of the drug reaching the cisternal area.[25]

The safety of intrathecal baclofen in pregnancy has not been established. One patient in our practice has completed two full-term pregnancies producing healthy infant girls by cesarean section delivery. Consistent with our experience, Delhaas and Verhagen describe the delivery of a healthy infant girl in a quadriplegic patient receiving intrathecal baclofen.[58]

An antagonist for baclofen is not yet clinically available, making dosing especially critical. Intravenous physostigmine may reverse the physiologic effects of overdose (see Chapter 6).

Opioids

Large concentrations of opioid receptors exist in the dorsal horn of the spinal cord, specifically in the marginal zone (lamina I) and substantia gelatinosa (lamina II). Morphine and other opioids bind to receptors on primary afferent terminals within the dorsal horn of the spinal cord,[59] inhibiting the release of various neurotransmitters, including substance P and others.[53,60] This inhibits pain transmission at the level of the spinal cord.[60,61] Morphine, hydromorphone, fentanyl, and sufentanil bind preferentially to mu (μ) opioid receptors, although others bind to delta (γ) or kappa (x) receptors. The potential advantage of opioids specific to non-μ receptors might be the lack of side effects seen with μ-receptor activity, such as respiratory depression.

Like baclofen, morphine is a relatively hydrophilic drug (Table 5.1). After an intrathecal injection of morphine, the average time of maximum activity at 20 to 40 minutes. The duration of action may extend as long as 24 hours.[34] Rostral flow is of concern with intrathecal use of opioids, especially with bolus administration, since the life-threatening side effect of respiratory depression is mediated by receptor binding to centers in the pons and medulla. Lumbar to cisternal concentrations of drug range from 4.6:1 (approximately 25%, similar to baclofen) to 7:1.[62,63]

Naloxone (Narcan) is an opioid antagonist that will bind preferentially to opioid receptors, and is useful when severe adverse events occur, particularly respiratory depression. Naloxone is given intravenously and should be reserved for truly emergency episodes since it may produce withdrawal in patients who have been chronically receiving opioids. Intrathecal morphine administration is associated with several adverse effects, some of which can be easily managed. Respiratory depression is the most feared effect and is, fortunately, rare when drug is administered within a standard dose range. The assessment and treatment of these adverse effects will be addressed in Chapter 7.

Safety

The toxicologic studies of intrathecal morphine administered in animals and humans indicate a lack of neuropathologic changes[62,64] when given chronically. Long-term use of intrathecal morphine delivered by implanted pump at numerous centers in the United States and Europe has proven to be safe, without neurologic damage.

Local Anesthetics

Local anesthetics, also called "membrane stabilizers," have been used alone or in combination with opioids for the relief of pain. Local anesthetics reversibly block sodium channels along the axon of the nerve, thereby inhibiting the action potential that propagates transmission of the pain impulse. The site of action of intraspinally administered local anesthetics is in the spinal cord as well as at the level of the spinal nerve roots in the intrathecal space.[65,66]

The most common intraspinally administered local anesthetic is bupivacaine (Marcaine, Sensorcaine),[67-72] although lidocaine and tetracaine have also been infused via the implanted pump. Bupivacaine is believed to differentially block pain fibers prior to altering other sensory modalities or motor ability.[73] The rationale for administering bupivacaine or other local anesthetics with opioids is the potential synergistic effect that has been shown to occur in animals given these drugs in combination.[74] The analgesic effect of these two agents given together may be greater than that seen with either drug individually. This might allow lower doses of each drug to be given, preventing or diminishing potential adverse effects seen with either of these agents. Additionally, patients with neuropathic pain might benefit from the addition of a local anesthetic.[69,72]

The side effects associated with intraspinal administration of local anesthetic are typically related to sympathetic blockade or vascular uptake of the drug.[69] The sympathetic nerve fibers adjacent to the spinal column are blocked during intraspinal administrated of local anesthetic, causing capillary dilation and pooling of blood.[66] This may result in a drop in blood pressure, potentially leading to orthostatic hypotension and falls when patients stand. Intravenous fluids should be available when initiating intraspinal local anesthetic therapy, particularly in dehydrated patients.

Higher doses of intrathecally administered local anesthetics lead to motor blockade, producing an inability to stand, ambulate, void, or defecate. Such high doses are not necessary to produce analgesia in the majority of patients and could cause significant morbidity. For example, four cases of cauda equina syndrome were reported after continuous infusion through external intrathecal catheters; however, it is not clear whether this was related to the drug or catheter.[75] Systemic absorption of the drug may lead to cardiac changes, including arrhythmias, and CNS toxicity, such as tremors or myoclonus. Patients may complain of tingling or numbness of the face as an early sign of systemic uptake.

The safety of local anesthetics administered chronically into the epidural or intrathecal space has not been established. Kroin and colleagues continuously infused intrathecal bupivacaine in dogs for periods of 3 to 16 weeks.[76] No damage was seen to the spinal roots, nor was any pathology noted within the spinal cord, providing evidence for the safety of this technique. However, lidocaine and tetracaine have not undergone this type of testing; thus toxicologic studies are needed prior to long-term use in humans.

Noradrenergic Agonists

Noradrenaline and related compounds are known to be involved in endogenous pain modulation. Attempts to mimic these endogenous systems have led to the use of intraspinally administered α_2-adrenergic agonists, such as clonidine. Clonidine and other α_2-adrenergic agonists bind to pre- and postsynaptic receptors in the dorsal horn of the spinal cord, inhibiting the release of substance P and subsequent firing within the spinal cord.[77] Current experience with this agent has largely been with epidural administration, although some investigators are examining the use of this agent given intrathecally. When administered epidurally in combination with opioids, there appears to be a synergistic analgesic effect of clonidine when compared with either drug given alone.[78]

Adverse effects noted with epidural administration of this drug include sedation, dry mouth, bradycardia, and hypotension.[77,79] Other α_2-adrenergic agonists, including tizanidine, which might have less hypotensive effect than clonidine, are being evaluated.[80] Although these agents are not yet available for clinical use, α_2-adrenergic agonists show promise as excellent analgesics when given spinally, and may provide particular benefit for patients with neuropathic pain syndromes.

Somatostatin

Somatostatin receptors are located in the dorsal horn of the spinal cord[81] and somatostatin appears to be an inhibitory transmitter in the spinal cord.[82] This led investigators to examine the possible role of somatostatin in modulating pain. Initial success with the intrathecal administration of native somatostatin in four patients with severe cancer pain[83] led to the use of the more stable analogue octreotide in cancer patients with severe pain unrelieved by oral opioids. Patients were treated for periods of 13 to 91 days with doses of 5 to 20 μg/h.[84] Pain intensity scores diminished, as did supplemental opioid doses. Although others have replicated these results,[85] the extraordinary cost of the drug (more than $20,000/year in the United States) precludes its use. Other somatostatin analogues are under study.

NMDA Antagonists

The N-methyl-D-aspartate (NMDA) receptor is involved in pain processing, particularly pain that is neuropathic in quality. NMDA antagonists have been shown to relieve pain when administered systemically but with resultant cognitive effects, such as hallucinations. This class of drugs includes phencyclidine (PCP) and is known to cause dissociative anesthesia. Spinal use might prove a reasonable method to administer these drugs directly to the site of action with little systemic delivery.

Caution is warranted, however. Although NMDA antagonists have been shown to reduce nociception when administered intrathecally in rats,[86] few safety and toxicity data are available regarding intraspinal use of these agents. Ketamine, an NMDA antagonist that has been used in anesthesia for many years, was shown to cause neurotoxicity in rabbits when given intrathecally, although the solutions used in this study also contained preservatives.[87] Conversely, a recent study of repeated intrathecal injections of ketamine in a rabbit model revealed an absence of neurotoxicity.[88] Future toxicity studies are necessary before ketamine and other NMDA antagonists are used intraspinally in humans for chronic administration.

■ CONCLUSION

Although baclofen and morphine are the only drugs currently approved for intraspinal use delivered via implanted infusion pumps, new agents are constantly being developed and tested. Understanding the pharmaco-kinetic properties of these agents will allow clinicians to appreciate how these drugs produce responses when given into the spinal space. This also provides the basis for clinical management of patients receiving these drugs.

6

Intrathecal Baclofen for Spasticity

Spasticity can be a serious complication of trauma to the spinal cord or other disorders that create damage within the spinal cord. Although affecting a small percentage of the population, spasticity can be devastating to the person experiencing it by limiting function, reducing mobility, complicating sleep, causing pain, and interfering with the quality of life. Spasticity management has included exercising and stretching programs, oral medications, and destructive neurosurgical procedures. A new, alternative treatment incorporates the use of an implanted pump which precisely delivers baclofen, through a catheter, directly into the intrathecal space. This treatment has proven to be extremely successful in reducing spasticity and is indicated for individuals with severe spasticity of spinal origin who have failed oral drug therapy. To fully comprehend the treatment of spasticity, one must understand the various definitions of spasticity as well as the physiology of this phenomenon and its interference with quality of life.

■ SPASTICITY

Definitions

Two definitions are commonly used to describe spasticity. The first definition by Wiesendanger, emphasizes the physiologic characteristics: "Spasticity is a movement disorder that develops gradually in response to a partial or complete loss of supraspinal control of spinal cord function. It is characterized by altered activity patterns of motor units occurring in response to sensory and central command signals which lead to co-contractions, mass movements and abnormal postural control."[89] The definition by Lance is more commonly used for clinical purposes:

"Spasticity is a motor disorder characterized by a velocity-dependent increase in tonic stretch reflexes (muscle tone) with exaggerated tendon jerks, resulting from hyperexcitability of the stretch reflex, as one component of the upper motor neuron syndrome."[90] A summary of these definitions relevant to both physiologic and clinical characteristics is found in Table 6.1.

The first definition emphasizes muscle incoordination and the occurrence of cocontractions in spasticity. During cocontractions both agonist and antagonist muscles are contracting, resulting in boardlike rigidity, extension or flexion of upper and/or lower extremities. Also fundamental to the first definition are mass movements and abnormal postural control. These are thought to be due to changes in motor control signals from supraspinal centers (the cortex, brainstem, and spinal cord) and local interneuronal changes within the spinal cord.

The second definition emphasizes tonic stretch reflexes, which can be measured by performing tests of range of motion. The velocity-dependent increase in tonic stretch reflexes, or muscle tone, is also key to this definition. The velocity-dependent nature of the reflexes refers to the more pronounced resistance as the exercises are performed more rapidly.

Regardless of the definition one accepts, the clinical picture is the same. Patients with spasticity cannot make smooth voluntary movements, and spasms of varying intensity interfere with many aspects of their lives. To better appreciate the clinical symptoms and treatment of spasticity, knowledge regarding motor control is essential.

Table 6.1. Physiological and Clinical Components
of Spasticity.

Physiological characteristics

- Loss of supraspinal control of spinal cord function causes spasticity
- Both sensory stimuli and central command signals can initiate spasticity
- Since several neural pathways and/or centers can be disrupted, activity patterns of motor units are altered (this is why spasticity can be different even in patients with identical diagnoses)

Clinical

- The onset is gradual
- Spasticity increases when increased velocity is exerted while doing ROM
- Stretch reflexes are typically hyperreflexive
- Spasticity can be identified by cocontractions, mass movements, and abnormal postural control

---

(Summarized as defined by Lance, 1980,[90] and Wiesendanger, 1991.[89])

Physiology of Motor Systems

The physiology of motor control is extraordinarily complex, and the mechanisms of spasticity are poorly understood. Table 6.2 lists several references that provide more in-depth discussions of motor control and the physiology of spasticity; however, for the purposes of this chapter, only a basic discussion will be provided.

Understanding the organization of the motor system is essential. The hierarchical arrangement of the motor control system begins with the highest level of control at the cerebral cortex, which projects its fibers directly into the brainstem and spinal cord (Fig 6.1). The basal ganglia and cerebellum affect motor control primarily through the cerebral cortex. With fibers from the cerebral cortex and the subcortical centers, neuronal fibers within the brainstem descend and terminate in the spinal cord. From the spinal cord, motor neurons project directly to the muscles, communicating information received from the supraspinal centers.

Of particular interest in motor control is the pyramidal tract because of its role in precise, voluntary movements. The pyramidal tract, also referred to as the corticospinal tract, descends from the cortex to the spinal cord. The fibers originate in the cortex, pass through the internal capsule, then continue downward through the brainstem, forming the

Table 6.2. References on Spasticity.

Ashby, P, McCrea D. **Neurophysiology of spinal spasticity.** In: Davidoff R, ed. *Handbook of the Spinal Cord.* New York, NY: Marcel Decker, Inc., 1987;119–143.

Lance J. The control of muscle tone, reflexes, and movement: Robert Wartenberg Lecture. **Neurology.** 1980;**30:**1303–1313.

Müller H, Zierski K, Penn R, eds. *Local-Spinal Therapy of Spasticity.* 1988, Berlin: Springer-Verlag; 1988:270.

Penn RD, ed. Neurological applications of implanted drug pumps. *Ann NY Acad Sci.* 1988;531–215.

Penn RD, Corcos DM. **Spasticity and its management.** In: Youmans JR, ed. *Neurological Surgery.* Philadelphia, Pa: W.B. Saunders Company; 1990:4371–4385.

Sindou M, Abbott R, Keravel, Y. *Neurosurgery for Spasticity: A Multidisciplinary Approach.* New York: Springer-Verlag; 1991.

Young RR, Delwaide PJ. Drug therapy: spasticity (first of two parts). **N Engl J Med.** 1981;304(1):28–33.

Young RR, Delwaide PJ. Drug therapy: spasticity (second of two parts). **N Engl J Med.** 1981;**304:**96–99.

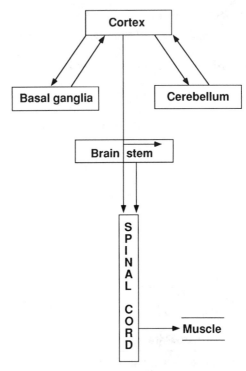

Figure 6.1. Simplified scheme of the hierar-
chial levels of motor control. (*Proposed by
McKeough.*[91])

pyramids of the medulla. Most of the pyramidal fibers decussate, or cross
to the opposite side, and descend in the lateral corticospinal tract. Those
that do not cross form the ventral corticospinal tract. A large portion of
the pyramidal tract fibers terminate in the intermediate regions of the
spinal cord gray matter. This region in the CNS is known to contain large
quantities of motor neurons.

The termination of fibers from the central motor pathways into the
motor neurons begins the branch of the peripheral nervous system. The
nerve impulses from motor neurons cause the skeletal muscle to contract.
In clinical practice, the terms upper motor neuron and lower motor
neuron are used to distinguish between the central motor pathways
(which generate commands from the higher center) and the lower motor
neurons (which transmit nerve impulses to the muscles).

Because the pyramidal fibers are important to movement, damage to
or interruption of these fibers leads to impaired movements, referred to

as an upper motor neuron syndrome. The clinical signs of upper motor neuron damage include initial flaccid paralysis followed by spasticity. Hyperreflexia, or abnormally brisk reflexes, occur because of the loss or altered input from pyramidal and other fibers that provide information from higher centers. For example, hyperreflexia can be seen when testing the patellar reflex. In the normal individual, when a reflex hammer is used to stretch the patellar ligament, the muscle is stretched, leading to a brief reflex muscle contraction. Stimuli from the muscle afferent neurons, as well as signals from the higher centers within the CNS, combine to orchestrate the response. When higher centers are damaged, or when damage occurs to the tracts that provide communication between the higher centers and the spinal cord, the normal controls are missing. This leads to an exaggerated response, known as hyperreflexia.

The upper motor neuron syndrome should be differentiated from lower motor neuron syndrome. The signs of lower motor neuron damage include weakness, muscle wasting, minute contractions within the muscles called fibrillations, and areflexia.

Clinical Characteristics of Spasticity

There can be great variability in the course of upper motor neuron syndrome; however, several characteristics are distinct. The onset of spasticity is gradual and is usually seen after an initial episode of flaccidity or loss of normal tone, occurring after spinal cord trauma or exacerbation of multiple sclerosis. After a time span ranging from days to weeks, spasticity develops and passively moving the limb leads to increased resistance and sometimes jerking, flexing, and/or extending of the extremities. Because of the velocity-dependent nature of the spasticity, the more rapid the exerted force, the more pronounced the response.

The velocity-dependent nature of spasticity distinguishes it from the rigidity seen in Parkinson's disease or the contractures that occur with disuse. In these conditions, rigidity is uniform. Muscle tone is increased in both agonist and antagonist muscle groups even with low velocity. Rigidity may be further divided into lead pipe rigidity, where resistance is smooth, or Parkinsonism cogwheel rigidity, in which a resistance fluctuates. In a patient with true spasticity, however, passive range of motion elicits increased resistance until the muscle suddenly relaxes, known as the clasp-knife phenomenon.

Assessment of Spasticity

Spasticity can be assessed by testing several reflexes and measurements that can be obtained to quantify movement related to spasticity. Clinicians must know how to properly test reflexes and use specific scales such as the Ashworth and other tools. These tests range from simple tools that can be used in any setting, to the more complex measurement that may require sophisticated mechanical devices.

Reflexes

The deep tendon reflexes initiate muscle contraction when the tendon is percussed. They are tested using a reflex hammer; the examiner strikes a specific tendon and notes the response (generally hyperactive in patients who exhibit spasticity). Responses are graded from 0 to 4, with 0 being no response and 4 being hyperactive (Table 6.3). The responses are commonly documented on a stick figure (Fig. 6.2).

Almost all muscles have deep tendon reflexes but the commonly tested ones are biceps, brachioradial, triceps, patellar, Achilles, and plantar reflex. Clonus that is associated with reflexes can be elicited most easily at the knee or ankle.

Biceps Reflex

Flex the patient's arm 45° at the elbow. Place your index finger on the patient's biceps tendon (located in the antecubital fossa) and strike the reflex hammer on your index finger. This produces contraction of the biceps and flexion at the elbow.

Brachioradial Reflex

Flex the patient's arm upward 45° with the hand slightly pronated. With a reflex hammer, tap the brachioradial tendon approximately 2 inches above the wrist. This produces contraction of the brachioradial tendon with a flexion movement at the elbow.

Table 6.3. Scale of Responses Used to Score Deep Tendon Reflexes.

Grade	Deep tendon reflex response
0	No response
1+	Sluggish or diminished
2+	Active or expected response
3+	More brisk than expected, slightly hyperactive
4+	Brisk, hyperactive, with intermittent or transient clonus

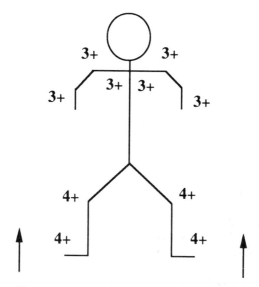

Figure 6.2. Documenting deep tendon reflex responses per "stick figure." Findings are typical of an upper motor neuron syndrome due to a spinal cord injury, for example.

Triceps Reflex

Flex the patient's elbow 90° while supporting the wrist with left arm. Tap the triceps tendon just above the elbow. This produces contraction of the triceps tendon with extension movement at the elbow.

Patellar Reflex (also known as the knee-jerk reflex)

The legs should be relaxed and flexed at 90°. Tap the patellar tendon just below the patella. This produces contraction of the quadriceps muscle and extension of the lower leg.

Achilles reflex (also known as the ankle jerk)

The patient is in a sitting position. The patient is asked to apply gentle plantar flexion onto the surface of the examiner's hand. Using the other hand, tap the Achilles tendon at the level of the malleoli. This produces contraction of the gastrocnemius muscle and plantar flexion of the foot.

Plantar reflex (also called the Babinski reflex)

Stimulate the lateral aspect of the sole of the foot using the metal end of the reflex hammer, in one brisk movement. The movement begins from the heel of the lateral side of the foot, curving across the ball of the foot to the medial side, causing flexion of the hallux. A normal response is flexion of the toes. An abnormal response, a Babinski, is dorsiflexion of the great toe with fanning of the other toes.

Clonus

Clonus can be induced in the ankle by a forceful dorsiflexion of the foot. Clonus is a hyperactive rhythmic movement between dorsiflexion and plantar flexion. This is commonly noted in patients with spasticity.

Measurement of Spasticity

The Ashworth Scale and spasm score are the most widely used tools to quantify spasticity and are the easiest to use (Table 6.4). Another method used to measure spasticity is slightly less sensitive, using the terms "mild,"

Table 6.4. Spasticity Assessment Scales.

Score	Criteria
Ashworth scale (rigidity/muscle tone)	
1	• No increase in tone
2	• Slight increase in tone, giving a "catch" when the affected part(s) is (are) moved in flexion or extension.
3	• More marked increase in tone but affected part easily flexed.
4	• Considerable increase in tone; passive movement difficult.
5	• Affected part(s) rigid in flexion or extension.
Spasm scale (Number of sustained flexor and extensor muscle spasms over 1-h interval)	
0	• No spasms
1	• No spontaneous spasms; vigorous sensory and motor stimulation results in spasms
2	• Occasional spontaneous spasms and easily induced spasms
3	• More than 1 but less than 10 spontaneous spasms per hour
4	• More than 10 spontaneous spasms per hour.

"moderate," or "severe" to rate resistance encountered with passive range of motion.

A more complex way to measure spasticity is by electromyelography (EMG). EMG can be used to rank or to compare different degrees of spasticity and normal muscle tone based on electric signals from affected muscles. It is common to apply force, or torque, to measure resistance to passive movement. This is done in a setting with specifically constructed devices. The information is especially useful in research studies on the nature of spasticity and its response to treatment.

Problems Related to Spasticity

The intensity of spasticity may change over time, and its functional impact varies with each patient. The following are the effects of spasticity seen in our own patient population:

Interference with sleep, causing daytime fatigue

Interference with activities of daily living

Interference with rehabilitation

Pain due to spasticity

Shearing of skin causing skin breakdown or pressure sores

Difficulty with mobility (including transfers and positioning)

Urinary incontinence due to a spastic bladder

Numerous conditions may lead to an increase in spasticity. For example, noxious stimuli may provoke increased spasticity. In a study of 60 male subjects with chronic spinal cord injury,[92] several triggers for increased spasticity are described. The most common is the urinary tract infection, which is very prevalent in this patient population. Other infections may also lead to increased spasticity, such as bone infections, which may take months to heal. Decubitus ulcers, whether infected or not, also increase spasticity. Bowel impaction, pain, and *disease progression* may also precipitate increased spasticity. Even a change of position, especially after a prolonged period in one position, or the physical stimulation of a light sheet can lead to spasticity. For some patients, a distended bladder, or merely emptying the bladder may generate increased spasticity. Several of our patients have undergone surgical procedures and have had increased spasticity for a short period of time. This may be attributed to physiological changes in response to surgery, or it may be stress-related, or both. Why these types of stimuli generate increased spasticity is unclear, but most produce increased sensory input to the spinal cord.

Psychosocial conditions such as a traumatic event or the serious illness of a significant other appear to cause increased spasticity, which is typically resolved when the stress is alleviated. In our experience, premenstrual syndrome has been shown to exacerbate spasticity. The underlying mechanism for this effect is also unknown.

The physiology of spasticity is complex and there may be little consensus regarding the underlying mechanisms; however, most clinicians agree that spasticity that interferes with daily living needs to be treated. Several treatment modalities may be instituted depending on the severity of spasticity, and will be discussed in the next section.

■ CURRENT METHODS OF TREATMENT

Physical Therapy

Spasticity may be treated initially with exercising and stretching programs. Active and passive range-of-motion (ROM) exercises may be effective in reducing the risk of contractures and may provide temporary relief of spasticity. When these programs become ineffective, pharmacologic interventions are added. Traditional antispastic agents such as baclofen, dantrolene sodium, and diazepam are commonly used.

Pharmacologic Management

Baclofen is the most commonly prescribed agent and is considered the most effective medication for reducing spasticity of spinal etiology while producing the fewest side effects.[93] Baclofen works by activating $GABA_B$ receptors that are located in the dorsal horn of the spinal cord.[11] These receptors are thought to limit the influx of calcium into the presynaptic terminals, resulting in a decreased release of excitatory neurotransmitters.[94] Unfortunately, when baclofen is administered orally, it does not easily penetrate the blood-brain barrier, since patients treated with 90 mg/d may show CSF concentrations below $0.1 \mu g/mL$.[95] Adverse effects most commonly reported with oral baclofen include: drowsiness, dizziness, weakness, and fatigue.

Diazepam works by enhancing presynaptic inhibition in the spinal cord by potentiating the postsynaptic effects of GABA.[96] Diazepam may produce tranquilizing, sedative, anticonvulsant, and skeletal muscle relaxant effects. There are receptors for this drug located throughout the brain and spine; however, the majority of the antispastic effect seems to occur at the spinal level.[94] Clinically, diazepam is most useful for patients with spinal cord lesions because it reduces painful flexor spasms.

Unfortunately, use of the drug is limited by centrally mediated adverse effects such as drowsiness, fatigue, and ataxia.

Dantrolene sodium acts directly on the muscle and inhibits the release of calcium from the sarcoplasmic reticulum and consequently inhibits activation of excitation-contraction coupling within the muscle fiber.[97,98] Dantrolene affects spasticity by diminishing the force of contraction.[94] This medication is useful for patients who have prolonged muscle contraction and who are not affected by the resultant decrease in voluntary muscle strength — that is, bedridden patients with quadriplegia or paraplegia. Because generalized weakness may occur, caution is needed when treating patients with concomitant myocardial disease or decreased pulmonary function.[99] Dantrolene sodium is not ideal for long-term use because of its association with hepatotoxicity.[100]

Other pharmacological agents used to control spasticity include clonidine and tizanidine. Clonidine is well known to clinicians as a centrally acting antihypertensive agent. This alpha-2 receptor agonist reduced tonic activity in the hindlimbs of paraplegic rats.[101] The mechanism of action of clonidine is unknown in reducing spasticity; however, one theory supports its occupying of alpha-2 receptor sites within the spinal cord, thereby decreasing motor responses. Donovan et al report 56% of patients with spasticity due to spinal cord injury benefitted from the drug; however, no effect was observed in 44% of the patients.[102] Unfortunately, clinical usefulness of this drug is limited owing to adverse effects such as postural hypotension, dizziness, drowsiness, and insomnia.[102]

The clonidine transdermal patch appears to be an effective treatment for spasticity after spinal cord injury. Weingarden and Belen report a positive antispastic response and minimal adverse effects using this mode of delivery.[103]

Tizanidine is an imidazoline derivative, closely related to clonidine. Its action on the alpha-2-adrenergic neurons of the locus coeruleus probably modulates tonic reflex activity. Clinical trials with oral tizanidine report efficacy in reducing spasticity in patients with spinal cord injury. Tizanidine is generally well tolerated. However, adverse effects include decreased heart rate, decreased diastolic pressure, infrequent sedation, and dryness of mouth.[104,105] Unfortunately, tizanidine is not FDA approved for use in the United States.

Electrical Stimulation

Chronic electrical stimulation of the CNS has been used to suppress spasticity and is attractive because it does not damage cord tissue, is relatively easy to perform, and is reversible. This surgical procedure can be only slightly invasive, employing percutaneous installation of wire leads into the epidural space by means of a puncture needle. It is thought that segmental reflexes are modified by activating inhibitory descending pathways or partially blocking excitatory pathways. Spinal cord stimulation does seem to reduce spasticity in some patients; however, long-term efficacy using this technique remains experimental.[106] Cervical stimulation has been tried, and results from controlled studies demonstrated no positive response.[107] The effect of cerebellar stimulation on spasticity in cerebral palsy was studied and initial reports demonstrated physical changes resulted from less spasticity.[108,109] Later, more carefully controlled studies confirmed no significant changes in spasticity and did not support its efficacy for this application.[110]

Intrathecal Agents

Two other intrathecal agents, both opioids, have been used to treat spasticity. Erickson et al reported that 1 to 4 mg of intrathecal morphine dramatically relieved pain and spasticity in several patients.[111] They assumed that spasticity is a combination of gamma and multisynaptic reflex activity and that the action of morphine disrupts the multisynaptic reflex arc. The continuous infusion of intrathecal morphine continues to be a successful alternative for relief of spasticity in some patients and has been used when patients develop tolerance to intrathecal baclofen. (See later section on tolerance.)

Intrathecal fentanyl is a second agent that has been used to successfully reduc espasticity. In a single patient who was resistant to chronically administered baclofen, intrathecal fentanyl reduced spasticity and produced no weakness or sedation.[112] Unfortunately, tolerance to this drug developed within 2 to 3 weeks of initiation.[112] The FDA has not approved intrathecal morphine or fentanyl for the application of spasticity, nor is fentanyl approved for use in implanted pumps. In fact, ancedotal evidence suggests that fentanyl may cause the SynchroMed pump to stall.

Invasive/Surgical Management

Invasive methods of controlling spasticity include ablative procedures and chemical neurolysis. Intrathecal alcohol or phenol in 5% glycerin is the most commonly used agent to destroy the reflex arc in patients whose spasticity is refractory to conventional methods. The greatest disadvantage of this procedure is the high risk of bowel or bladder sphincter dysfunction and voluntary motor weakness.

The orthopedic approach to treating spasticity consists of surgically releasing fixed contractures, muscle- and tendon-lengthening procedures, and open neurectomies. Neurectomies and tendon-cutting procedures eliminate the possibility of future recovery with voluntary movement. Releasing procedures eventually fail when the underlying disorder of increased muscle tone is not treated.[112]

Numerous destructive neurosurgical procedures have been performed for intractable spasticity. Procedures such as selective peripheral neurectomies, various rhizotomies, myelotomies, and the DREZ procedure (dorsal root entry zone) are being done, but are not uniformly successful. Each of these procedures has its own rationale. However, they all involve disrupting the reflex arc that drives motor neurons. Unfortunately, these procedures are irreversible and can cause weakness and sensory loss. The selective dorsal rhizotomy and the percutaneous radiofrequency foraminal rhizotomy are two procedures that create lesions, but only to the nerve roots causing muscle contraction, thus preserving cutaneous and joint sensation. Ablative surgical procedures are generally indicated when spasticity is severe and all other attempts for management have failed.

A new method for reducing intractable spasticity is the chronic infusion of intrathecal baclofen through an implanted delivery system. This treatment modality has proven to be effective in dramatically reducing spasticity in multicenter clinical trials conducted in the United States and Europe.[19,114–118] The advantages of this treatment include the following:

1. Baclofen is delivered directly to the site of action in the spinal cord, resulting in a dramatic clinical effect.

2. The implanted delivery system permits a constant CSF level of the drug.

3. Systemic side effects are rare.

4. Doses can be precisely adjusted according to individual needs.

5. The surgical procedure is nondestructive.

6. The treatment and delivery system is not permanent, allowing future options for spasticity control to be explored.

There are two distinct disadvantages of this treatment:

1. A long-term commitment is required from patients.

2. The mechanical delivery system may fail and need subsequent repair involving surgery.

Despite the obvious disadvantages, most patients suffering with severe, disabling spasticity have few options and thus consent to long-term treatment.

■ BENEFITS OF REDUCED SPASTICITY

Spasticity can have a positive or negative effect on a patient's quality of life and ability to function. Not all spasticity is bad; in some persons a mild degree of spasticity is an advantage for performing activities such as transferring and ambulating. In contrast, severe uncontrollable spasticity causes pain, interferes with function, and often interrupts sleep. The programmability of an implanted device allows doses of baclofen to be precisely titrated, resulting in reduced spasticity and optimal function.

Function

Function may be compromised when spasticity is severe and uncontrolled. Patients often report pain associated with spasms and difficulty performing activities of daily living. Lower extremity flexor and extensor spasms prohibit patients from transferring, getting in and out of bed, sitting in their chairs, and, for some patients, driving. Patients with severe hip adductor spasms have difficulty performing urinary catheterization and hygiene procedures. Ambulating may be more difficult when lower-extremity flexor spasticity interferes with smooth, voluntary movement (Fig. 6.3). Intractable spasticity may result in joint dislocations, contractures, and pressure sores, which increase a person's risk for further immobility and infection. When spasticity is controlled, patients are more comfortable, daily care and range of motion exercises are easier to perform, and function may be optimized.[115,117,119] The severely impaired patients benefit when correct body alignment can be restored and they can be easily turned and repositioned (Fig. 6.4).

Bladder Function

The extent of baclofen's effect on the genitourinary system is not completely understood, but it appears to have a substantial influence on function. This effect is variable depending on dose, spinal pathology and baseline bladder and urethral function.[120] Urodynamic studies support baclofen's effect on increasing bladder capacity and decreasing detrusor-sphincter dyssynergy[121] (Fig. 6.5). Intrathecal baclofen has been shown to be effective in reducing urethral pressure, although not consistently.[122] Some patients benefit by simplifying their bladder management programs, for example, from indwelling catheters to intermittent catheterization procedures.[115,119,120,122] Others benefit by staying drier between catheterization procedures and reported ease in performing the technique.[115,119] These improvements occur in parallel to the reduction in

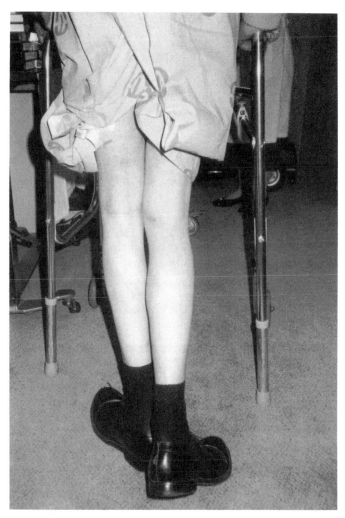

Figure 6.3. 52-year-old male diagnosed with spastic quadriplegia secondary to cerebral palsy. Ambulating is difficult
because of severe hip adduction contributing to a scissorslike
gait.

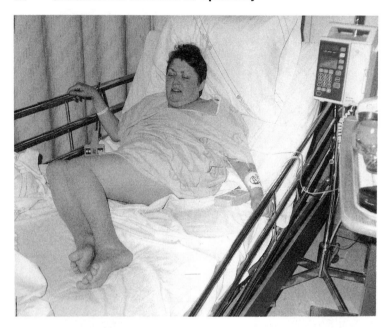

Figure 6.4. (A) Positioning of the legs before intrathecal baclofen. (B) Difficulty sitting in motorized chair because of spasms causing extension at the hips. (C) Two hours after an intrathecal baclofen bolus of 75μg, full range of motion can be initiated easily and the legs can be extended at a greater angle.

spasticity. It is likely that higher doses of baclofen could produce an even greater effect on the bladder, but higher doses are not indicated because of potential overdose and hypotonia.

Bowel Function

Intrathecal baclofen does not appear to have a consistent effect on defecation. Subjective reports by a few patients indicate that high doses of intrathecal baclofen caused frequent and urgent defecation; however, most patients state that baclofen does not effect their bowel routines.

Pain

The majority of patients receiving intrathecal baclofen experience an increase in comfort. Pain specifically associated with frequent muscle spasms or persistent rigidity can be reduced and even eliminated in most cases. Taira et al. report five patients who experienced central pain after

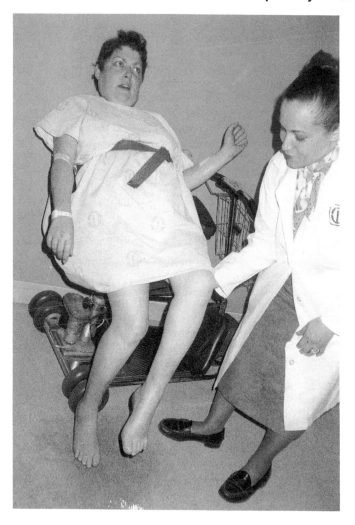

Figure 6.4(B)

stroke, achieved pain relief after a bolus of intrathecal baclofen.[123] Neuropathic or deafferentation pain, often characterized as burning or tingling, does not seem to be relieved by intrathecal baclofen. This may reflect a different pathophysiology.[116]

Sleep

Sleep disruption is often a major source of discomfort for patients suffering with severe spasticity. Patients receiving intrathecal baclofen

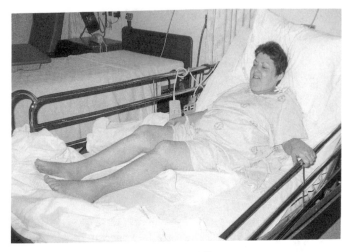

Figure 6.4(C)

have reported fewer nocturnal awakenings from spasms and have reduced arousal-related EMG activity.[119,124] Baclofen is thought to have a minimal direct effect on the sleep centers because of the low cisternal concentration, and its effect is attributed to reduced muscle spasms.

Mobility

Improved mobility is demonstrated in a variety of ways and depends on the patient's underlying disease process, level of lesion, rehabilitation programs, and individual motivation and determination. Although few of our patients are capable of ambulating, those who can walk benefit when the speed and duration of their gait are increased. Generally, these patients remain dependent on assistive devices to ambulate, but they may upgrade from a walker to crutches or canes. Nonambulatory patients benefit when they can transfer and stand with greater confidence and ease or independently locomote in their wheelchairs. Severely impaired patients with extreme muscle weakness may be mobilized with less effort when resistance from spasticity is reduced.

Upper-extremity weakness and spasticity further limit the patient's mobility. Intrathecal baclofen may have a minimal effect on upper-extremity spasticity. Kroin and Penn report a lumbar to cisternal concentration gradient of 4:1.[25] It seems logical that a small amount of baclofen at the cervical level could produce a slight antispastic effect at corresponding spinal segments. A few patients reported decreased spasticity and a relaxed feeling to the upper extremities after a bolus dose was administered. However, patients receiving baclofen at a low contin-

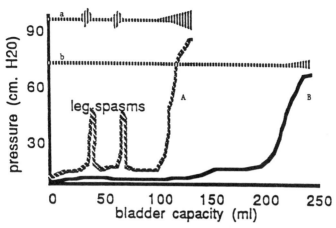

Figure 6.5. Sphincter EMG and cystometrogram tracing from a 27-year-old male with spasticity secondary to a T_9 fracture after trauma. (a) Sphincter EMG data and (A) cystometrogram tracing showing a transient rise in intravesical pressure associated with leg spasms and a detrusor reflex at 100 mL of filling before baclofen. (b) Sphincter EMG and (B) cystometrogram tracing 2 years after his injury with initiation of intrathecal baclofen showing minimal EMG activity and a detrusor response at 225 mL of bladder filling. (Reprinted with permission by Frost et al. Intrathecal baclofen infusion: effect on bladder management programs in patients with myelopathy. *Am J Phys Med.* 1989; 68(3):112–115.)

uous rate do not experience a dramatic clinical effect to their upper extremities. High doses may be necessary to produce an effect but are generally not indicated because of inadvertently causing lower extremity hypotonia and cerebral adverse effects.

Quality of Life

The effect of reduced spasticity from intrathecal baclofen on quality of life is being investigated. Preliminary results from a pre/post trial are encouraging (Gianino and York, preliminary results). Reduced spasticity may indirectly influence one's self-esteem. Returning to work, attending school, driving, and becoming more involved with family responsibilities and community activities are examples of activities that affect quality of life.

Neurophysiologic Function

Latash et al. investigated the neurophysiological effects of intrathecally administered baclofen by monitoring mono- and polysynaptic reflexes and muscle responses during attempts at voluntary movement in six patients with severe spinal spasticity.[125] Intrathecal baclofen was found to profoundly depress both mono- and polysynaptic reflexes; in addition, improved voluntary muscle control as reflected by more selective activation of different muscle groups was present in three patients.[125] Unfortunately, the level of voluntary activation in all three patients was too low to permit useful function. Findings from this study are significant because they support baclofen's selective inhibitory action on different motor paths.

■ PATIENT SELECTION

Health professionals from many disciplines who are skilled in performing neurologic assessments are key in identifying patients likely to benefit from intrathecal baclofen therapy. Patients are considered for intrathecal baclofen based on the following criteria:

1. The patient must be diagnosed with severe spasticity of spinal origin such as that seen with MS or SCI.
2. The patient must be refractory to oral baclofen or experience adverse effects from antispastic medications.
3. The patient must respond positively to a trial injection (bolus) of intrathecal baclofen of $\leq$ 100 μg. A positive response to a bolus consists of a significant decrease in muscle tone or frequency and/or severity of spasms. It is recommended to use the Ashworth and spasm scales to determine a change (Table 6.4).[126,127] A reflex assessment may also be helpful.

Patients who are not appropriate candidates for this therapy include:

1. Those who are allergic or hypersensitive to oral baclofen.
2. Those who require a substantial amount of muscle tone to sustain their upright posture or balance in locomotion.
3. Patients with other implanted programmable devices (e.g., pacemaker) because cross-talk between the two devices can inadvertently change the prescription.

Caution is advised when treating patients with the following conditions:

1. Impaired hepatic or renal function.
2. Women of childbearing age who are pregnant or not using birth control methods because of the unknown effects on the fetus.
3. Nursing mothers.
4. Patients operating dangerous machinery.

Many psychosocial factors influence patients' eligibility and compliance with the long-term treatment, and these should be considered when selecting patients. Patients with significant psychiatric disorders or those with a history of substance abuse may be noncompliant with refill schedules, and, more importantly, inaccurate dosing may result because of concomitant drug effects with baclofen. It is believed that alcohol may produce an additive effect with intrathecal baclofen, as reported by many patients.[128] Cocaine's effect with baclofen remains unknown. Patients and their families experiencing significant stress or dysfunction may be noncompliant with the treatment. Inadequate transport services and large geographical distances from the health care provider should be considered, but these problems are not as restricting since more high-tech home health nurses have been educated in providing these services. Although chronic intrathecal baclofen therapy has proven to be cost-effective, a lack of financial resources or exhausted insurance benefits may hinder a patient's ability to receive and/or maintain the therapy for a long period of time.

Other Motor Disorders

The success in treating spasticity from spinal etiology has generated interest in the drug's effect on spasticity secondary to other motor disorders. Table 6.5 identifies patients with a variety of motor disturbances who have had a bolus injection of intrathecal baclofen and their responses. Intrathecal baclofen appears to be effective for some individuals with spasticity secondary to cerebral palsy.[118,129,130,131,132] Albright et al. report that a continuous infusion of intrathecal baclofen is particularly useful for patients who require some spasticity to stand and ambulate because doses can be titrated precisely to each individual's needs.[131] Penn et al. report two of six patients with cerebral palsy who were not ideal candidates for intrathecal therapy because a dramatic loss of trunk and lower extremity muscle tone interfered with function.[129] Both groups of investigators report that baclofen did not affect athetoid movements that were present in some of the patients. A multicenter study of intrathecal baclofen's effect on spasticity from cerebral palsy is currently being conducted in the United States. Patients are selected and classified by stringent criteria. Preliminary results have been encouraging.

Intrathecal baclofen has also been dramatically successful in treating patients with Stiffman syndrome. These individuals suffer with debilitating rigidity and spasms that affect their extremities and axial musculature. Two patients who failed high-dose oral diazepam achieved dramatic spasticity control and excellent pain relief.[133] Conversely, Ford and Fahn report on one patient diagnosed with late-stage Stiffman

Table 6.5. Intrathecal Baclofen Injection for a Variety of Movement Disorders.

Diagnosis	Patient age/gender	Maximum bolus injection	Response	Comment
Wilson's disease	24 male	100 μg	No response	
Anoxic encephalopathy	39 female	75 μg	No response to UEs	Weaker LEs
	17 male	100 μg	No response	
	36 male	100 μg	No rsponse	
Primary lateral sclerosis	71 male	100 μg	(+) response	More difficult to ambulate
	62 male	300 μg	No response	
	60 male	75 μg	(+) response	More difficult to transfer
	48 male	200 μg	No response	
Cerebral palsy	11 male	50 μg	(+) response	Withdrew R/T decreased truncal tone
	11 male	75 μg	(+) response	Improved function
	45 male	75 μg	(+) responseq	Improved comfort
	52 male	75 μg	(+) response	Slightly improved function
	13 female	75 μg	(+) response	Decreased truncal tone
	42 male	75 μg	(+) response	Difficulty with transfers

Traumatic brain injury	18 female	75 µg	(+) response	Withdrew R/T meningitis
	42 female	100 µg	(+) response	Improved comfort/function
	18 male	100 µg	(+) response	Improved comfort/function
Perioperative cerebral infarction	34 female	100 µg	(-) response	No implant R/T geographical distance
Lathorism	55 male	50 µg	(+) response	Dramatic effect, improved function
Stiffman syndrome	40 male	75 µg	(+) response	Partially controlled movements
Dystonia generalized	53 male	100 µg	(+) response	Developed tolerance
hemi	36 male	100 µg	(+) response	Decreased foot movement
focal	40 male	75 µg	(+) response	Decreased posture/gait
R leg	37 female	100 µg	(+) response	Increased comfort; ambulation easier
focal	60 male	100 µg	(+) response	
Shy-Drager syndrome	48 female	75 µg	(-) response	
Painful legs moving toes syndrome	44 female	75 µg	(+) response	Decreased foot movement
Probable spondylosis	75 female	75 µg	(+) response	Decreased pain and mass reflexive response

(Continued)

Table 6.5. (*Continued*)

Diagnosis	Patient age/gender	Maximum bolus injection	Response	Comment
Cervical myelopathy secondary to neurofibroma	71 male	75 μg	(+) response	Mild functional improvement
Cervical hydromyelia	60 female	50 μg	(+) response	Poor balance and gait, weaker extremities
White matter neurodegenerative disease — unknown origin	52 male 76 male 64 male	75 μg 75 μg 100 μg	(+) response (−) response (−) response	Initial weakness, no implant R/T geographical distance

(Adapted with permission by Penn et al.[127])

Syndrome not responding to intrathecal baclofen.[134] The reason for this disparity is unclear.

Intrathecal baclofen appears to be effective for a variety of dystonic disorders. Narayan et al. report one patient with axial dystonia being successfully treated.[135] Penn et al. report five patients with different types of dystonia achieving varied effects.[129] One patient with generalized dystonia achieved only subtle improvement in his gait and movement. Two patients with focal foot dystonia experienced decreased foot movements and improved gait. One patient with a hemidystonia initially responded to the treatment but gradually lost the effect within about 6 months of treatment.[129]

Patients with fixed dystonic posture and rigidity secondary to anoxic encephalopathy, Shy-Drager syndrome and Wilson's disease did not respond to an intrathecal baclofen injection.[129] In contrast, a small number of patients with spasticity due to traumatic brain injury experienced reduced spasticity, enabling greater ease of care and positioning.[118, 129]

Because the number of patients treated with intrathecal baclofen for a variety of motor disorders other than spinal spasticity is limited and their responses are inconsistent, additional clinical trials should be conducted. Larger samples may more accurately represent the response seen in these patient groups. The vast majority of these patients have failed oral therapy and are desperate for relief. The same factors affecting the classic candidates (patients with MS and SCI) such as the expense and commitment to a long-term therapy must be weighed against the potential benefit.

Patients selected to receive the treatment require a comprehensive physical and functional assessment at baseline and throughout the long-term phase. The Ashworth and spasm scales are useful for quantifying spasticity, and a reflex assessment is also recommended. Because patients with severe spasticity often have further neurologic impairment that interferes with the function of many systems, an organized functional assessment helps track progress or deterioration (Table 6.6).[128] Functional deterioration correlates with the progression of the disease process, particularly in MS, and is not a consequence of the chronic baclofen therapy.

Patient education is critical; patients and their families need to understand information about the risks of the procedure, the benefits of the therapy, and the technology involved in the delivery system. A patient-teaching checklist is provided to help clinicians ensure thorough instruction (Table 6.7). The amount of information may be overwhelming at first, and needs to be repeated periodically throughout all phases of the therapy. Verbal information and written materials are essential. Appendix 1 is an example of a booklet specifically developed for patients who will receive intrathecal baclofen. Appendices 3.3, 5, and

Table 6.6. Physical/functional assessment.

Impaired physical mobility
- purposeful movement of extremities
- vasomotor instability
- spasticity
- restricted movement
- difficulty with transfers
- difficulty with locomotion
- use of assistive devices
- use of splints (inhibitory or supportive)
- inability to propel a wheelchair

Total or partial self-care deficit
- ability to feed self
- ability to dress/groom self
- ability to grasp or grip tools and utensils
- ability to transfer onto toilet/commode
- ability to transfer onto shower chair/bathe
- ability to manage bowel program
- ability to manage bladder program

Cognitive deficit
- confusion/disorientation
- judgment
- memory
- problem solving

Sleep pattern disturbance
- interrupted sleep
- difficulty in initiating sleep
- use of medications to induce sleep
- inadequate amount of sleep (day and night)

Chronic pain (dysesthetic vs spasticity related)
- associated irritability/fatigue
- avoidance of certain activities
- withdrawn behavior
- use of inappropriate measures for relief
- factors that induce pain

Sexual function
- limitations
- impotence

Impaired skin integrity
- presence of shearing forces
- presence of pressure sores

Sensory deficit
- alterations in tactile sensation
- proprioception
- inability to sense sources of potential danger

Altered bowel elimination
- constipation/diarrhea
- extent of control
- type of program used for control

Altered urinary elimination
- extent of control
- type of catheterization
- diversional route
- frequency of infections

Altered cerebral tissue perfusion
- orthostatic hypotension
- dizziness

Altered peripheral tissue perfusion
- edema
- enlarged veins, venous stasis
- history of PE/DVT
- numbness, tingling
- decreased arterial pulses

Impaired breathing pattern
- phrenic nerve pacers
- bradypnea
- degree of thorax expansion, symmetry
- respiratory quality, rate, and rhythm

(Continued)

Table 6.6. (*Continued*)

Impaired verbal communication	High risk of aspiration
• presence of articulate speech • ability to make gestures • quality of voice	• alterations in the ability to chew and swallow • need to support head in an upright position while eating or drinking • need to clear the upper and lower airway • Control of tongue and mouth muscles

(Reprinted from *Rehabilitation Nursing.* 1993; 18(2): 105–113, with permission of the Association of Rehabilitation Nurses, 5700 Old Orchard Road, First Floor, Skokie, IL 60077–1057. Copyright 1993 Association of Rehabilitation Nurses.)

6 are additional references that may be helpful for patients and their caregivers. Refer to Chapter 4 for further instructions regarding pre- and postoperative teaching.

■ SCREENING PROCEDURES

Patients are selected to receive a trial of baclofen based on the inclusion criteria, physical and functional assessments, and potential benefits from the therapy. Most patients are admitted as inpatients into hospitals where monitors and emergency equipment are readily accessible. Experienced practitioners may elect to screen patients in outpatient settings. Regardless of the setting, the screening trial is conducted in an environment that is fully equipped and staffed to monitor the respiratory and cardiovascular systems and care for patients. The screening trial is indicated only for patients free from infection because the presence of an infection may increase spasticity and therefore skew the response to the bolus (trial) injection.

The screening trial consists of the following steps:

1. Prepare a 50-μg bolus of intrathecal baclofen to be administered via lumbar puncture. (To dilute the 500 μg/mL solution of baclofen, add 9 mL of sterile, preservative-free sodium chloride to 1 mL of 500 μg/mL baclofen to obtain a total of 10 mL.)

2. Draw into a sterile syringe 1 mL of the diluted baclofen to equal 50 μg/mL. (In the future, ampules containing small doses adequate for a trial injection may be commercially available from the manufacturer.)

3. By LP or spinal catheter, inject 1 mL of the prepared solution (50 μg/mL) as the initial dose, and discard the remaining solution. (Using external spinal catheters for serial trial doses may increase

Table 6.7. Patient-teaching checklist (prescreening).

I. Drug effect

    ✓ Fewer adverse effects
    ✓ Dramatic spasticity reduction
    ✓ Potential benefits/risks

II. Cost

    ✓ Pump
    ✓ Hospitalization (surgery)
    ✓ Surgeons' fees
    ✓ Maintenance (drug, refill procedure, evaluation, future diagnostics tests)

III. Screening

    ✓ Location (in hospital)
    ✓ Lumbar puncture (bolus injection)
    ✓ Monitoring devices
    ✓ Peak effect and duration
    ✓ Possible adverse effects

IV. Surgery

    ✓ Incision location
    ✓ Anesthesia used
    ✓ Length of procedure
    ✓ Length of hospital stay
    ✓ Risks of surgical procedure

V. Delivery system (pump, catheter, programmer)

    ✓ Pump feature (size, alarms, bacteriostatic filter)
    ✓ Catheter placement
    ✓ Flexible programming options for precise dosing
    ✓ Potential system complications

VI. Refill procedure/follow-up appointments

    ✓ Frequency of refills
    ✓ Length of time during office visit
    ✓ Evaluations
    ✓ Sterile refill procedure
    ✓ Dose adjusting

---

the patient's risk for infection. Also, intrathecal bolus injections may be difficult to perform in the presence of spinal stenosis, scoliosis, and scar tissue; hence, fluoroscopy may be required to confirm intrathecal drug placement.)

4. Attach the appropriate monitoring devices to the patient—i.e., cardiac-apnea monitor or pulse oximetry. (Monitoring the patient

with this equipment is optional but recommended because central adverse effects from the bolus are possible.)

5. Monitor the patient's vital signs and assess for adverse effects (Table 6.8) and the response to the drug using the Ashworth and spasm scales in approximately 1-hour intervals. This monitoring should continue for at least 6 to 8 hours:

baclofen's onset of action:	1 to 2 hours
peak action:	2 to 4 hours
duration of action:	4 to 8 hours

6. If the patient demonstrates a positive response to the bolus dose (significant decrease in muscle tone and/or spasms; generally a 2-point decrease on the Ashworth or spasm scale), the pump may be implanted.

7. If the patient does not achieve a positive response to the 50 μg bolus dose, repeat the procedure using 75 μg or 1.5 mL of the prepared solution 24 hours after the first screening bolus.

8. If the patient demonstrates a positive response to the trial, the pump may be implanted.

9. If the patient does not achieve a positive response to the 75 μg bolus dose, repeat the procedure, for the last time, using 100 μg, 24 hours after the second bolus dose. (Patients who do not respond to a 100 μg bolus are not candidates for the therapy. Bolus doses exceeding 100 μg are not recommended.)

Patients vary in their sensitivity to baclofen. Most patients do not experience adverse effects, while others may experience severe adverse effects. Table 6.8 lists the most commonly reported adverse effects during the screening trial. Special attention is needed to recognize the signs and symptoms of an overdose:

Drowsiness

Dizziness

Lightheadedness

Somnolence

Visual disturbance

Slurred speech

Respiratory depression

Seizures

Rostral progression of extreme hypotonia

Loss of consciousness

Table 6.8. Most frequently reported adverse effects during the screening procedure.

Drowsiness
Dizziness/lightheadedness
Hypotension
Weakness, lower extremities
Nausea/vomiting
Hypotonia

Refer to the section on patient management and dosing for specific guidelines in treating an overdose.

■ PATIENT MANAGEMENT

Successfully managing patients over a long period of time combines the art and science of intrathecal baclofen administration. Our goals are to administer the medication safely and maintain its efficacy over a long time. The success of the therapy depends on precisely adjusted doses programmed for each individual's needs. Because intrathecal baclofen is commercially approved for use through the SynchroMed pump, this section will focus on patient management and relevant interventions using this delivery system.

A comprehensive spasticity assessment is fundamental for patient management. Dose adjustment is based on a combination of several factors including the patient's subjective statements and an objective spasticity assessment. The Ashworth and spasm scales are helpful for quantifying spasticity, and a basic reflex assessment may supplement data obtained from the spasticity assessment. Also, the patient's ability to function is significant when adjusting doses of baclofen, particularly when patients require some muscle tone to function optimally.

The onset and duration of spasticity may provide clues that baclofen doses are subtherapeutic or that a system malfunction is suspected. Generally, spasticity that is persistent and occurs abruptly is associated with a pump or catheter malfunction. On the other hand, a gradual onset of spasticity may indicate that the dose is subtherapeutic. The frequency and intensity of nociceptive stimuli must be considered in a spasticity assessment; for example, sharp pain accompanying operative procedures, gallbladder attacks, and kidney stones provides stimuli that trigger spasticity. The patient's mental status and concomitant psychosocial events are variables that may influence spasticity control. Subjective reports by patients correlate extreme stress with a temporary increase in spasticity. Lastly, the drug delivery system must be checked for accuracy, as a small catheter kink will result in a pump reservoir fluid discrepancy.

Postoperative Management

The continuous infusion of baclofen is started during the time of surgery. The initial daily dose is determined by doubling the screening dose that produced an effect. For instance, if a patient positively responded to a 50 μg bolus during screening, a continuous infusion of 100 μg per 24 hours would be programmed. If the effect of the screening dose exceeded 12 hours, then patients may begin on that dose or lower doses. This prolonged effect is most frequently seen in patients who are very sensitive to the drug or who ambulate. During the immediate postoperative period, doses should not be changed more frequently than every 24 hours. This time frame is needed for the drug to diffuse into the spine and reach a steady state. Also, antispastic medications and drugs used during the operative procedure or for postoperative pain may add to baclofen's effect. Patients remaining on oral antispastic medications should have them gradually discontinued over several weeks, because their abrupt withdrawal can lead to serious adverse effects. Specifically, rapid withdrawal of oral baclofen has been associated with hallucinations, seizures, and hypothermia.[136-138]

The immediate postoperative period may not be the ideal time to achieve an optimal dose. Consecutive dose adjustments are usually required after patients are discharged and return to their home environments and daily routines. Patients are initially very sensitive to the drug and respond dramatically to small increases and decreases. A few patients have experienced poor voice quality, bladder incontinence, and generalized weakness during the first and second postoperative days. These transient adverse effects were successfully treated by decreasing the continuous infusion. One male reported difficulty initiating an erection for approximately 1 week after intrathecal baclofen was started. Fortunately, this problem resolved soon afterward without any dosing intervention. Similar cases have been reported and corrected by decreasing intrathecal baclofen.

A less frequently encountered situation is when spasticity is not relieved during the postoperative period. At times, initial continuous doses are too low and afford minimal spasticity relief. Generous dose increases approximating 20% to 30% of the previous dose may be required to achieve adequate control. Occasionally, postoperative complications—for example, a catheter tear—may result in inadequate spasticity relief despite consecutive, substantial dose increases. The following case report presents a postoperative catheter malfunction that complicated dose finding and describes the sequence of events that followed.

Case Report

J.B. was a 12-year-old male who was referred for treatment of intractable spasticity due to a SCI at birth. J.B. sustained a C_5, T_{4-5}, and brachial plexus injury at birth as he descended from a front breech presentation. He was taking 60 mg of oral baclofen per day which did not control his spasticity, and further increases in dose produced drowsiness which interfered with his ability to concentrate at school. After a successful response to the screening intrathecal bolus dose of 50 μg was achieved, J.B. and his parents decided to have the drug pump surgically implanted to facilitate continuous delivery. J.B.'s pump was programmed to deliver 120 μg/d, using 500 μg/mL concentration.

On the first postoperative day J.B. experienced no change in his spasticity (average Ashworth score 4.5, spasm score 3). A 150 μg bolus was programmed. J.B. had no response to the bolus. On the second postoperative day J.B.'s spasticity remained uncontrolled, and he complained of a headache. His intrathecal baclofen dose was increased to 216 μg/d. On the third postoperative day J.B.'s spasticity was slightly better (average Ashworth score 3.5, spasm score 2). His intrathecal baclofen dose was increased to 300 μg/d. J.B. continued to complain of a slight headache particularly when sitting, and pain around his back incision. His surgical incisions were assessed and appeared to be healing well without redness or swelling.

On the fourth postoperative day J.B. was discouraged about his lack of spasticity relief and annoying headache accompanied by nausea every time he sat up. His intrathecal baclofen dose was significantly increased to 600 mg/d and he finally began to respond a few hours later with decreased rigidity and spasms (average Ashworth score 2.5, spasm score 1). When J.B.'s response to the increased dose was evaluated, his incisions were assessed and he had a moderate amount of swelling localized beneath the back incision and directly over the pump. Even though J.B.'s spasticity was well controlled, he continued to have persistent headaches and nausea. J.B. was taken to the operating room and had the spinal catheter explored. CSF was escaping from a small hole that was noted proximal to the lumbar insertion site. After the spinal catheter was replaced, J.B.'s remaining surgical course was unremarkable. He achieved excellent spasticity relief and was discharged on a dose of 209 μg/d.

Discharge

Explicit discharge instructions must be provided to the patient, their family, and caregivers. Patients are particularly receptive to new information during this time when the surgery is over. Discharge instructions should include the following content: follow-up appointments, wound care, activity restrictions, concomitant medications, a schedule for "tapering" antispastic medication, and recognizing emergent situations and properly accessing the health care system for assistance. Refer to Table 4.1 for an example of written discharge instructions. Figures 6.6 and 6.7 are emergency cards provided by Medtronic, Inc, that should be reviewed and given to each patient. These cards contain specific information including the drug, overdose and treatment, and correctly accessing the pump.

Long-Term Patient Management

Patient management consists of physical examination, pump refills, adjusting doses, psychosocial assessments, and referrals. Most patients return to clinics or hospitals for long-term management; however, home care nurses are becoming skilled at providing these services and are often consulted for refilling and adjusting doses for severely debilitated patients who are bedridden. The frequency of follow-up care depends on the patient's dose, response to the dose, adverse effects, and drug stability. Baclofen is stable in the pump for at least 90 days. The refill interval is the number of days until the pump reaches the low reservoir alarm level.

The low-reservoir alarm is generally programmed to sound when 2 mL of drug remains in the reservoir. The low reservoir alarm may be postponed or programmed to sound at any mL amount depending on the clinical situation.

The refill interval may be calculated by the following equation:

(1) Calculate usable reservoir volume

Usable reservoir volume = reservoir volume
                          − low reservoir alarm volume

(2) Calculate refill interval

$$\text{Refill interval} = \frac{\text{usable reservoir volume} \times \text{drug concentration}}{\text{daily dose}}$$

Example: Calculate the refill interval for a patient receiving 400 μg baclofen per day with a 2000 μg/mL concentration and a low-reservoir alarm set at 2 mL.

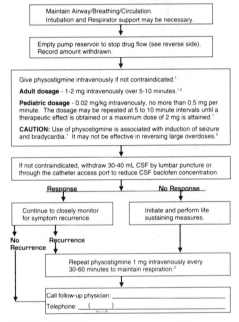

EMERGENCY PROCEDURE
FOR Lioresal® Intrathecal (baclofen injection) Overdose

SynchroMed Infusion System:

Programmable drug pump implanted in abdominal wall connected to an intrathecal catheter. Implanted pump contains an 18mL drug reservoir and may have more than one port (a reservoir port and a catheter access port).

Symptoms:

Drowsiness, lightheadedness, dizziness, somnolence, respiratory depression, seizures, rostral progression of hypotonia and loss of consciousness progressing to coma.

Actions:

Maintain Airway/Breathing/Circulation.
Intubation and Respirator support may be necessary.

↓

Empty pump reservoir to stop drug flow (see reverse side).
Record amount withdrawn.

↓

Give physostigmine intravenously if not contraindicated.[1]

Adult dosage - 1-2 mg intravenously over 5-10 minutes.[1,2]

Pediatric dosage - 0.02 mg/kg intravenously, no more than 0.5 mg per minute. The dosage may be repeated at 5 to 10 minute intervals until a therapeutic effect is obtained or a maximum dose of 2 mg is attained.[1]

CAUTION: Use of physostigmine is associated with induction of seizure and bradycardia.[1] It may not be effective in reversing large overdoses.[2]

↓

If not contraindicated, withdraw 30-40 mL CSF by lumbar puncture or through the catheter access port to reduce CSF baclofen concentration.

Response ↓ **No Response**

| Continue to closely monitor for symptom recurrence. | Initiate and perform life sustaining measures. |

No Recurrence / **Recurrence** ↓

Repeat physostigmine 1 mg intravenously every 30-60 minutes to maintain respiration.[2]

↓

Call follow-up physician: _____
Telephone: ____(____)_____

1 Physostigmine manufacturer's package insert.
2 Müller-Schwefe G., Penn R.D. Physostigmine in the treatment of intrathecal baclofen overdose: report of three cases. *JNeurosurg*, August, 1989; 71:273-275.

Figure 6.6. Emergency procedure for intrathecal baclofen overdose. *(Card provided by Medtronic, Inc.)*

(1) Calculate usable reservoir volume

$$18 \text{ mL} - 2 \text{ mL} = 16 \text{ mL}$$

(2) Calculate refill interval

$$\frac{16 \times 2000}{400} = 80 \text{ days or } 11.4 \text{ weeks}$$

EMERGENCY IDENTIFICATION

I am on a medication called **BACLOFEN.** It reduces my muscle spasticity. The medication is stored in a drug pump implanted in my abdomen and is delivered through a catheter into my spinal column.

Signs of a drug reaction or overdose are:

- Lightheaded and dizzy, progressing to extreme drowsiness or sleepiness
- Breathing becoming very slow and shallow (less than 10 per minute)
- Unconscious or unable to awaken

Actions if severe symptoms of drug reaction or overdose appear, check:

- **Airway** ▶ Open Airway
- **Breathing** ▶ Look and listen for breaths—if none, give breaths into victim. Call your emergency number for help.
- **Circulation** ▶ Check for a pulse—if none, give cardiac massage (CPR). (If you do not know how to give CPR call emergency number immediately.)

Seek Emergency Medical Attention:

1. Give them baclofen **Emergency Procedure** card.
2. Have them empty the pump.
3. Have them call your doctor at _____

Figure 6.7. Wallet size emergency card to be carried by patients receiving intrathecal baclofen. *(Card provided by Medtronic, Inc.)*

As the pump nears the 2 mL volume remaining in the reservoir, some patients tend to experience an increase in spasticity. In these cases, low-reservoir alarms may be set to alarm sooner (e.g., at 3 or 4 mL). The pump manufacturer warns that infusion rates decrease approximately 15% when the reservoir volume drops below 2 mL.

Dosing

Proper dosing is critical for successful long-term management. The goal of dose titration is to provide optimal spasticity control without compromising function using the lowest possible dose. Baclofen doses vary considerably between patients. There has not been any consistent correlation between daily doses and factors such as the following:

1. Amount of oral baclofen
2. Age
3. Sex
4. Height/weight
5. Severity of spasticity
6. Diagnosis
7. Level of injury
8. Duration of spasticity

Baclofen doses are usually adjusted during follow-up visits when the pump is refilled. We recommend using the Ashworth and spasm scales to score spasticity and serve as a guide for adjusting doses. Generally, doses are increased in 10% to 40% increments when excessive muscle tone and spasms return (Table 6.9). In most cases, an increase of 1 or 2 points on either scale indicates a 10% to 20% increase in dose. Larger increases of 30% to 40% are indicated when spasticity scores have increased by 3 to 4 points. Table 6.10 lists data from 25 patients at their follow-up appointments pertaining to dosage adjustments. The mean dose increase is 16%; the mean dose decrease is 13%.

Table 6.9. Guidelines for increasing intrathecal baclofen doses.

Ashworth/spasm score	Percent increase/decrease
↑ 1 point	10–20%
↑ 2 points	20–30%
↑ 3 points	20–40%
↑ 4 points	30–40%*

*Assess for patient-related or delivery system complication.

Table 6.10. Patient Data: Percent Increase or Decrease.

Patient sex	Age	Dx	Mos. receiving baclofen	Dose	Average Ashworth	Average spasm	% ↑ or ↓ or no change	Comment
F	28	SCI	105	980	1	0	—	Content
M	48	MS	8	75	2.25	2	↓ 15%	MS exacerbation on Solumedrol
M	34	SCI	6	170	1	0	—	Content
F	63	MS	105	576	1	0	—	Content
F	31	MS	1	98	1	0	↓ 15%	LEs weak; can't transfer
F	50	MS	48	446	4	1	↑ 30%	Work-up for system malfunction
F	22	SCI	11	550	1.5	.5	—	Content
F	60	SCI	42	192	1	0	—	Content
M	45	MS	66	450	2	2	↑ 30%	Rigid
F	31	MS	1	114	1	0	↑ 10%	Painful spasms
F	50	MS	48	613	1	0	↓ 20%	Dizziness, poor voice production
F	37	MS	9	47	1	0	↑ 5%	Spasms sitting in one position
F	61	MS	58	1200	3.5	1	—	Content
F	52	MS	44	250	1	0	↓ 5%	Too flaccid
F	30	MS	32	92	1	0	—	Content
F	50	MS	74	1200	2	1	—	Content
F	59	MS	20	700	3.25	1	↑ 5%	Empty pump
F	46	MS	75	550	1.75	1	↑ 10%	Easily induced spasms
F	35	MS	59	425	1	0	—	Content
F	43	MS	44	600	4	3	↑ 20%	Septic—in hospital
F	31	MS	100	207	1	0	—	Content
F	37	MS	2	120	1	0	—	Content
F	41	MS	6	120	1	0	↓ 10%	Too flaccid
M	38	SCI	6	637	1	0	↑ 15%	Upper-extremity spasms
M	51	SCI	68	659	1	0	—	—

If patients do not satisfactorily respond to an increase in dose, a system malfunction or exacerbation of an underlying disease should be suspected. These possibilities should be ruled out prior to increasing the dose further. However, there are exceptions when increased baclofen doses are temporarily warranted for patients suffering with uncontrolled spasticity due to other physical problems, such as severe infections. The healthcare provider must remember to make every attempt when the acute medical problem has resolved to lower the patient's dose back to the previous levels that provided adequate spasticity relief.

Patients very sensitive to the drug who experience hypotonia and other adverse effects seem to tolerate smaller dose adjustments of 10% to 15% as their spasticity changes. Baclofen doses may be decreased when some muscle tone is needed to enhance optimal functioning, such as transferring, or when adverse effects such as drowsiness, lightheadedness, or slurred speech occur. Patients capable of ambulating tend to require lower daily doses, preserving some muscle tone needed for this activity. These patients can be challenging to manage because they often require frequent, subtle dose adjustments before a therapeutic balance of muscle tone can be achieved (Fig. 6.8).

Doses vary considerably and range between 12 and 1500 μg/d (Fig. 6.9). The majority of patients are maintained on doses between 200 and 700 μg/d. Few patients actually require doses less than 50 μg or more than 1200 μg/d. Data from long-term studies are needed to provide information about dose requirements over time versus tolerance. Ninety percent of our patients who have been receiving baclofen for more than 8 years are maintained on doses averaging 320 μg/d.

Patients typically develop a physiological tolerance to the drug between 4 and 24 months or longer, requiring a gradual increase in dose. Doses tend to stabilize after this time (Figs. 6.10, 6.11) It is not unusual for patients to request a change in dose each time they are due for a refill. Precisely titrated doses stabilize over time, after incisions have healed and activity is optimized.

Upper-extremity spasticity is a concurrent symptom present in some of our patients. Because a small amount of baclofen may ascend to the cervical level in the subarachnoid space, it seems likely that the upper extremities would be minimally affected. Few patients have been treated by increasing the amount of intrathecal baclofen. Unfortunately, increasing the dose to the higher levels that may control upper-extremity spasticity may produce hypotonia in the lower extremities or central adverse effects. This situation is particularly evident in patients who ambulate. These patients have been treated with small doses of oral baclofen in addition to their intrathecal dose. Small, systemic doses of baclofen may afford some spasticity relief to the upper extremities; however, caution is needed when adjusting doses using this combination.

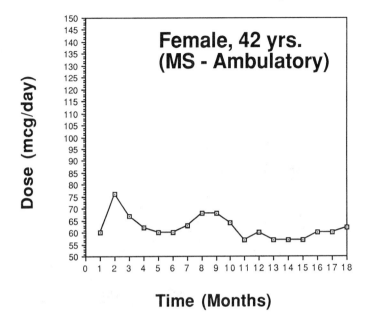

Time (Months)

Figure 6.8. Graph illustrating the dose escalation pattern in a 42-year-old female diagnosed with multiple sclerosis who ambulates. Doses are adjusted monthly, in small increments, needed to maintain a proper balance of muscle tone enabling independent ambulation.

Intrathecal baclofen's effect on the reproductive system remains unknown. A few male patients reported difficulty initiating or maintaining an erection. One patient had difficulty initiating an erection immediately after the therapy was initiated. He was discharged on a daily dose of 280 μg and fortunately, this problem resolved within 1 week without any intervention. Another male reported inconsistency in initiating erections. His daily baclofen dose was 330 μg. He was successfully treated by lowering his dose to 230 μg/d; however, he had to put up with the nuisance of increased spasticity. We have not encountered any detrimental effects from intrathecal baclofen on the female reproductive system. Two females have successfully conceived and delivered healthy infants while receiving the drug.

Infusion Modes

Simple-Continuous/Simple-Complex Cycle
Programming dose adjustments is possible through a variety of infusion modes employed by the SynchroMed pump. The simple-continuous and

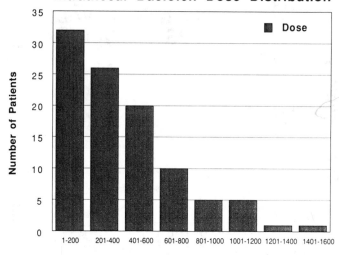

Figure 6.9. Bar graph representing intrathecal baclofen dose distribution from patients at Rush-Presbyterian-St. Luke's Medical Center, Chicago, Ill. The majority of patients are maintained on daily doses <600 μg per day. (N = 102 pts.)

the continuous-complex cycles are most frequently used (Fig. 6.12). Most patients achieve successful control of spasticity by a simple continuous cycle (the same amount of drug is administered every hour). Others require different amounts of drug during the day or night to either enhance functions or attain maximal spasticity control. The latter group is best managed by a complex cycle (the drug is delivered continuously, but at different rates in a repeated series of specified steps). Generally, a 24-hour pattern is programmed. The complex cycle may be ideal for those who (1) experience greater spasticity at night, interfering with sleep; (2) require some amount of muscle tone to sustain upright posture, transfer, ambulate, and other activities during the day; and (3) experience severe spasticity at various times during the day induced by activity.

The complex cycle consists of a series of 10 possible steps from which to program different doses. Usually, two to three steps comprise the cycle which is timed over 24 hours.

The most common complex cycle consists of two steps that deliver more drug at night, allowing a sound, uninterrupted sleep. Patients specify the timing of the cycles based on when they sleep and awaken. Delivery rates are programmed to increase or decrease approximately 2 hours before the time specified by the patients, allowing time for the drug

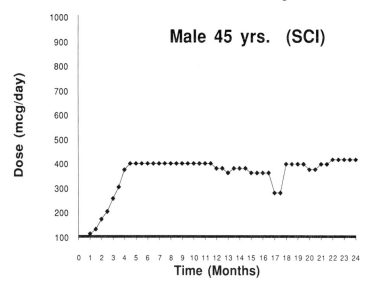

Figure 6.10. Dose escalation pattern of one male whose dose stabilized at 400 µg/d after 4 months after initiating intrathecal baclofen therapy.

at the increased rate to diffuse into the spine. This time delay is based on studies from bolus doses leading to a full clinical effect. When the drug is infusing at a continuous rate, we expect this time delay to be actually longer. The night dose is initially determined by increasing the day dose 20%; however, further increases may be needed to achieve a satisfactory night dose. Refer to the SynchroMed Infusion System Clinical Reference Guide provided by Medtronic Inc. for specific programming instructions.

Patients whose spasticity is difficult to control may benefit from a periodic bolus of drug delivered in addition to continuous rate. This dosage prescription is programmed infrequently and is particularly useful for patients who notice trends of increased spasticity occurring during the same time of day which is unrelieved by a simple or complex continuous infusion. A bolus of drug generally elicits a favorable response in addition to a continuous infusion. The complex-cycle delivery mode is used to facilitate this prescription. Caution is needed when programming even small boluses along with a continuous infusion because adverse effects or overdose may result.

Periodic Bolus (Bolus Delay)

The periodic bolus or bolus delay mode delivers a prescribed dose at specified intervals. We have not used this delivery mode to manage

DOSE ESCALATION PATTERNS

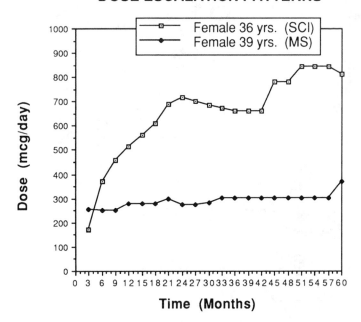

Time (Months)

Figure 6.11. Dose escalation patterns of two patients receiving intrathecal baclofen over 5 years. The baclofen dose stabilized at 24 months for the patient with SCI. Also, she required a substantial increase in drug at 42 months. In contrast, the dose for the patient with multiple sclerosis stabilized at 3 months. *(Reprinted with permission from Gianino.[139])*

patients with spasticity because constant drug CSF levels are preferred, resulting in uniform spasticity control. Again, the potential for overdose exists with multiple bolus delivery.

Bolus

Lastly, the bolus mode allows a large dose of baclofen to be administered rapidly. This mode is most often used for determining lack of efficacy related to subtherapeutic dosing or a delivery system problem. For example, bolus doses of either 50 or 75 μg are programmed at their fastest rates with the intent to produce a dramatic decrease in spasticity. Patients must be assessed 1 to 2 hours after the bolus was programmed for a change in spasticity. If the patient positively responded to the bolus, the delivery systems performance is probably intact, and higher doses may be

INFUSION MODES USED FOR PATIENT MANAGEMENT
(Patient's represented at RPSLMC, Chicago, IL)

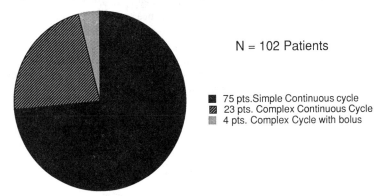

N = 102 Patients

■ 75 pts. Simple Continuous cycle
▨ 23 pts. Complex Continuous Cycle
▧ 4 pts. Complex Cycle with bolus

Figure 6.12. The simple-continuous cycle is most commonly used for managing patients. The complex cycle is useful for managing patients who experience greater spasticity at various times during a 24-hour period. A few patients require a bolus of baclofen at specified times, in addition to a complex cycle.

needed to control the spasticity. If the patient does not respond to a bolus, then a system complication such as a catheter disconnection must be suspected.

The bolus mode may be used for two other applications. Depending on the clinical situation, a bolus may be programmed for patients with uncontrolled spasticity due to a completely empty pump at the time of a refill. Also, a bolus is needed when changing drug concentrations to "bridge the gap" between higher and lower drug concentrations present in the pump tubing and catheter.

Changing Concentrations

Intrathecal baclofen, manufactured by Ciba-Geigy, Switzerland, is commercially available in two different concentrations and is labeled as Lioresal Intrathecal. The drug is available in 500 μg/mL and 2000 μg/mL concentrations. The 500 μg/mL concentration is prepared in a 20-mL ampule labeled "10 mg/20 mL." The largest available concentration is prepared in a 5-mL ampule labeled "10 mg/5 mL." Four ampules (5 mL) are needed for an 18 mL volume consisting of 2000 μg/mL. At present, the baclofen injection refill kit contains all the supplies needed to refill the pump safely, including the drug.

Any concentration less than 2000 μg/mL may be easily prepared by diluting the available formulations with preservative-free sodium chloride for injection. The most commonly used concentrations are 500 μg/mL, 1000 μg/mL and 2000 μg/mL. A concentration of 250 μg/mL is easily prepared for patient requiring very small daily doses of baclofen (e.g., 35 μg/d), but the majority of patients begin with a 500 μg/mL concentration and are at doses greater than 50 μg/day. Drug concentrations are determined by the daily amount, the refill frequency, and most importantly, the minimal flow rate specified by the pump manufacturer ensuring accurate drug infusion. Pump models 8611H, 8615, and 8615s are used for administering intrathecal baclofen and require a minimal flow rate of 0.096 mL/24 h. The flow rate is calculated by:

$$\frac{\text{Daily dose}}{\text{Concentration}}$$

Pump flow rates must be considered when selecting concentrations. Drug concentrations are increased as daily doses escalate and allow a longer refill interval. Table 6.11 may be used as a reference for determining minimal flow rates.

Whenever drug concentrations or solutions are changed, the remaining old drug in the pump tubing and catheter must be accounted for to prevent over- or underdosing the patient. When changing from a low concentration to a high concentration, the patient may be temporarily underdosed, unless the amount of drug remaining in the pump tubing and catheter is programmed to infuse at an equivalent rate over a calculated amount of time. Underdosing will result when the pump is programmed to deliver the same amount of drug at a higher concentration. The pump rotor will turn at a slower rate to deliver the dose. Eventually, the pump tubing and catheter will be "primed" with the new, higher concentration, and the patient will then be receiving the actual prescribed daily dose. The opposite scenario is true for patients changing from a lower to a higher concentration; however, serious events result from overdose.

To avoid under- or overdosing a patient, a "bridge bolus" is calculated to account for the volume of drug remaining in the pump tubing and catheter at the "old" concentration. The amount of drug to give as a "bridge bolus" is determined by:

Volume of drug in the pump tubing × new drug concentration

After the amount of bolus is calculated, the duration of time over which it infuses is then calculated by:

$$\frac{\text{Old drug concentration} \times \text{volume in pump tubing and catheter}}{\text{New hourly rate}}$$

Table 6.11. Sample: Lioresal® Intrathecal
(baclofen injection) Daily Dose Requirements,
Concentration and Flow Rates*

Patient daily dose (μg)	Concentration (μg/mL)	Minimum flow rate (mL/day)
25	250 (dilution nec.)	0.1
50	500	0.1
100	500	0.2
150	500	0.3
200	500	0.4
200	2000	0.1
250	500	0.5
250	2000	0.125
300	500	0.6
300	2000	0.15
400	2000	0.2
500	2000	0.25
600	2000	0.3
700	2000	0.35
800	2000	0.4
900	2000	0.45
1000	2000	0.5

*Assumes 18-mL reservoir refill volume.
(Reprinted with permission by Medtronic.[136])

(Refer to the SynchroMed Infusion System Clinical Reference Guide for a table used to determine volume in pump tubing and catheter and details on how to safely program a "bridge bolus.")

Reservoir Rinse

In addition to performing a bridge bolus it is recommended that a reservoir rinse be performed twice to dilute the remaining drug in the pump reservoir dead space. The dead space contains approximately 2 mL of drug that cannot be removed by emptying the pump. If changing to a lower concentrated solution, failure to perform a reservoir rinse will result in a drug concentration greater than intended, leading to risk of overdose.

A reservoir rinse is performed by emptying the pump of the original drug and refilling it with the appropriate volume of preservative-free sodium chloride for injection. Repeat this step to further dilute the solution remaining in the pump reservoir dead space.

Adverse Effects

Patients vary in their sensitivity to intrathecal baclofen. Some patients experience virtually no adverse effects, but a few may experience severe adverse effects. Table 6.12 lists the most frequently reported adverse effects from monitored clinical trials in the United States. The incidence of adverse effects can be listed according to when they occur, including the screening, dose titration, and maintenance phases. The titration phase is defined as the period of time from initial pump implant to 2 months following. The maintenance phase is generally considered to be the 2-month period after pump implant.

Hallucinations have been reported by patients after abrupt withdrawal from intrathecal baclofen. Also, sudden cessation may result in a hyperactive state characterized by uncontrolled spasms and increased rigidity accompanied by anxiety, confusion, hyperthermia, diaphoresis, and rapid respirations.[136] Patients often describe their spasticity during these times as being worse than the spasticity experienced before initiating the therapy. Interestingly, seizures have been reported from patients who have abruptly withdrawn or overdosed from intrathecal baclofen.[137,138,140] Baclofen's effect on the seizure threshold remains unknown. Caution is needed when discontinuing or interrupting therapy; baclofen doses should be gradually lowered to prevent complications such as these from occurring.

Drug Interactions

There is inadequate experience with the use of intrathecal baclofen in combination with other oral medications to predict specific drug interactions. Alcohol and other CNS depressants may have an additive effect with intrathecal baclofen and produce hypotonia, drowsiness, slurred speech, and incoordination. The combination of antihypertensives and high doses of intrathecal baclofen can potentially lower blood pressure, so caution is warranted with dose titration and careful blood pressure monitoring. Corticosteroids such as prednisone and Solu-Medrol, commonly administered to patients with MS exacerbations, seem to potentiate baclofen's ability to produce hypotonia. In such cases, doses of intrathecal baclofen may need to be significantly decreased until the course of steroid therapy is completed and spasticity recurs.

Table 6.12. Incidence of Most Frequent Adverse Events in Prospectively Monitored Clinical Trials.

	Number of patients reporting events		
Adverse event	N* = 244 screening[†]	N = 214 titration[‡]	N = 214 maintenance[§]
Drowsiness	13	11	18
Weakness, lower extremities	1	11	15
Dizziness/lightheadedness	6	5	12
Seizures	1	4	11
Headache	0	3	9
Nausea/vomiting	3	5	3
Numbness/itching/tingling	2	1	8
Hypotension	3	0	5
Blurred vision	0	2	5
Constipation	0	2	5
Hypotonia	2	3	2
Speech slurred	0	1	6
Coma (overdose)	0	4	3
Lethargy	1	0	4
Weakness, upper extremities	1	0	4
Hypertension	1	2	2
Dyspnea	1	2	1

*N = total number of patients entering each period.
[†]Following administration of test bolus.
[‡]Two-month period following implant.
[§]Beyond 2 months following implant.
(Drug Labeling Insert, Courtesy of Medtronic, Inc, Minneapolis, Minn.)

Physical and Psychological Factors

There are several physical and psychological factors that tend to interfere with baclofen's efficacy. Patients with MS who have had an exacerbation of their disease present with insidious uncontrolled spasticity along with other neurological manifestations, namely weakness. If patients are not treated with steroids, a substantial increase in their baclofen dose may be necessary. For patients treated with steroids presenting with hypotonia, a significant decrease of baclofen may be temporarily needed. Unfortunately, patients with MS and SCI are susceptible to infections, including urinary tract infections, upper respiratory infections, or infected pressure sores, leading to an increase in spasticity. Other pathological conditions such as fractures, gallbladder disease, and stroke may also increase spasticity, making dosing of baclofen difficult. Extremely stressful events may be additional factors that seem to interfere with baclofen's efficacy. Patients presenting with these conditions must have their underlying disease treated first. Baclofen doses may be temporarily increased approximately 10% to 40%, but these and larger increases are generally inadequate in providing sufficient spasticity relief during these unique situations. If the dose of baclofen is increased, every attempt must be made to lower the patient's dose to previous therapeutic levels after the disease process has resolved.

Overdose

Special attention must be given to recognizing the signs and symptoms of overdose and when it is most likely to occur. Overdoses most commonly result from the following situations:

Accidentally filling the sideport or access port rather than the drug reservoir (model 8615-only).

Inaccurate programming.

Changing from a high to low concentration without using a bridge bolus.

Administering bolus doses.

Programming continuous dose increases greater than 40% to 50% at one time. This situation is particularly true for patients sensitive to baclofen.

Manually filling the spinal catheter with baclofen, using a needle during the surgical implant or revising procedures.

Unfamiliarity with microgram dosing units and inappropriately using milligrams instead, which are used for the oral preparation.

Use of concomitant medications such as diazepam.

Conducting catheter patency studies without accounting for the amount of medication present in the catheter.

The majority of overdoses are caused by bolus doses. The sudden rostral spread in the CSF is presumed to be the reason why baclofen boluses can result in overdose. A few patients report mild sedation associated with the supine position. The supine position may also enhance the rostral distribution of baclofen in the CSF.

The following case study describes a situation where overdose occurred while troubleshooting for a patient-related versus delivery system complication.

Case Study

P.L., a 41-year-old female, had a pump implanted for a continuous infusion of baclofen to treat her intractable spasticity. She sustained an incomplete C_7 fracture following an accident. Her postoperative course was unremarkable; she was discharged and maintained on a dose of 275 μg/day. Approximately 2 years later, P.L. complained of increased spasms along with itching, a tingling sensation all over, shaky voice, and emotional instability. An X-ray revealed a catheter kink proximal to the pump, which was surgically revised to restore patency. A few days later, P.L. complained of a dull headache, blurry vision, and flushing and was found to be hypotensive. Her baclofen dose was decreased by 20% to (220 μg/d), and a complex cycle was programmed for more drug during the night and less drug during the day. A couple of weeks later, P.L. presented with more spasms (average Ashworth score 2.5; spasm score 3) and requested an increase in the daytime dose. An increase was administered totaling 253 μg/d. Two days later, P.L. called with concerns about her drowsiness, slurred speech, and blurry vision, which warranted a decrease in dose to 230 μg/d.

For 2 months P.L. continued to have symptoms of a mild to moderate overdose each time her dose was increased, but could not achieve adequate spasticity relief. P.L. experienced disabling spasms which prohibited any independence using her upper extremities, and her torso was violently thrusted outward from her wheelchair. Again, X-rays were done and revealed proper catheter placement, inserted at L_{4-5} with the tip at approximately T_{11}. An indium-111 DTPA flow study was then conducted in the hospital to analyze baclofen flow in the CSF. Indium-111 DTPA was injected into the pump, mixed with the remaining baclofen, and programmed to infuse slightly faster. The intent for increasing the flow rate was to clear the pump tubing and catheter of the "pure" baclofen, allowing the baclofen mixed with contrast material to reach the spine.

Approximately 6 hours after the rate was increased, P.L. became drowsy. Soon afterward, she was transported to the nuclear medicine department for a follow-up scan when she reported blurry vision and had slurred speech. By the time the scan was complete, she was confused (trying to get out of the cart) and had garbled speech. P.L. was rushed to her room for continuous monitoringand eventually became somnolent and difficult to arouse. There were no corresponding changes in her vital signs. At that time 1 mg physostigmine was mixed with 30 cc 0.9%

sodium chloride and set to infuse intravenously over 10 minutes. P.L. showed no response and could not be fully aroused. Another 1 mg physostigmine was administered over 5 minutes and P.L. began to wake up. She required no further physostigmine and her drowsiness gradually improved. She continued to be closely monitored and had no changes in her vital signs.

It was calculated that P.L. received 150 μg of baclofen over 2 hours, which resulted in an overdose. Her indium-111 DTPA flow study showed baclofen present at the cisternal level, which indicates normal, rostral flow. P.L. was treated by having her spinal catheter repositioned with the tip resting at L_3. This level is generally not recommended to achieve a therapeutic effect; this case is an exception. Her remaining postoperative course was uneventful and she achieved adequate spasticity relief without central adverse effects on a continuous dose of 250 μg/day.

As this case illustrates, overdoses may occur abruptly or insidiously, and treatment is based on their severity. Overdoses occurring insidiously are generally mild and characterized by symptoms such as drowsiness, dizziness, lightheadedness, hypotonic nausea, and vomiting. On the other hand, a severe overdose may occur suddenly and may be manifested by drowsiness, confusion, loss of consciousness progressing to coma, visual disturbances, slurred speech, hypotonia, respiratory depression, and seizures.

Mild overdoses may be treated by simply decreasing the patient's dose. To date, there is no specific antidote for reversing overdoses of intrathecal baclofen. However, intravenous physostigmine has been successfully used to reduce central effects, namely drowsiness and respiratory depression.[141] Guidelines for treating an overdose include:

1. Stop the drug infusion and empty the residual baclofen from the pump reservoir.

2. ADULT DOSE: Administer 1 to 2 mg intravenous physostigmine over 5 to 10 minutes.
   PEDIATRIC DOSE: Administer 0.02 mg/kg intravenous physostigmine, no more than 0.5 mg per minute intervals until a desired effect is obtained or a maximum of 2 mg is administered.

3. Physostigmine should be administered very slowly (0.2 to 1 mg/min) to prevent seizures from occurring.[142,143] Assess for change in vital signs and neurologic status.

4. For the adult, doses may be repeated in 1-mg increments at 30 to 60-minute intervals in an attempt to maintain adequate respiratory function and level of consciousness. Physostigmine is short-acting, with an elimination half-life of 20 minutes, so repeated doses may be needed.[144]

5. Physostigmine is ineffective in reversing large overdoses; patients may require intensive care including respiratory support.

(Refer to Fig. 6.6, a convenient algorithm for recognizing and treating an overdose.)

Caution is advised when administering intravenous physostigmine because its use has been associated with bradycardia, cardiac conduction abnormalities, and seizures. The benefit of using physostigmine must be weighed against the risk of adverse effects. An alternative treatment requires a lumbar puncture to withdraw 30 to 40 mL of CSF to reduce the CSF baclofen concentration; however, timing is a critical factor with this intervention. If the CSF is not withdrawn soon after the overdose is detected, a significant amount of the drug may have already ascended to the cisternal level, causing severe central effects. Delhaas and Brouwers report five of seven overdose events requiring a combination of initial management with intravenous physostigmine followed by CSF withdrawal needed to improve respiratory function and level of consciousness.[145] Saltuari et al report one case of severe overdose (accidental intrathecal bolus of 10 mg) not responding to a physostigmine dose totaling 14 mg.[146] In this case 30 mL of CSF was removed, and the patient began breathing spontaneously 48 hours afterward. Overdoses may be difficult to reverse; however, most cases may be prevented by complying with safety standards.

Pump Replacements

Patients receiving intrathecal baclofen over a long period of time will eventually require pump replacement due to a low battery. The lithium battery contained in the pump lasts approximately 3 to 5 years or 44 months with infusion rates of 0.5 mL/d.[16] Longevity is related to the flow rate over time. Patients maintained on doses with corresponding flow rates of 1 to 1.5 mL/d will need their pumps replaced sooner than patients whose flow rates are less than 1 mL/d. The "low battery" alarm will sound when the battery depletes its energy source and will be indicated on the screen of the portable programmer after the pump is interrogated by the telemetry wand.

Replacing pumps due to low battery is not considered an emergency unless the battery is known to be low for several weeks and/or the patient is experiencing signs of withdrawal. Some patients experience greater spasticity when the battery is low. The pump manufacturer recommends that pumps be replaced as soon as possible because accurate infusion is not guaranteed. Depending on the clinical situation, pump replacements may be performed as an outpatient procedure.

■ TOLERANCE

Tolerance, also known as tachyphylaxis, can be frustrating to both patients receiving intrathecal baclofen therapy and their clinicians. Not only may the patient experience distress from increased spasticity, but tolerance is not easy to diagnose and the treatment may be troublesome. In fact, several problems we initially diagnosed as tolerance were actually delivery system complications related to holes in the catheter. The underlying mechanisms of tolerance are unclear, and assessment may be confounded by changes in the patient's physiological state or by system complications. One method of treating tolerance is with a drug holiday, although frequent drug holidays may be needed once tolerance is diagnosed.

Theories

The mechanisms of tolerance to baclofen, where increasing doses of drug are needed to maintain the original effect, are uncertain. Theories regarding tolerance to baclofen include possible changes at the $GABA_B$ receptor level or intracellular changes. Recent evidence suggests that tolerance to baclofen is related to changes at the receptor level.[147] Down-regulation (a decrease in the number of receptors) may occur after repeated drug delivery, or a decrease in the affinity of the receptor to the drug may be responsible. Studies conducted by Kroin et al. support the down-regulation theory,[148] where the number of $GABA_B$ receptors are decreased, causing baclofen to become less effective because there are fewer receptors on which to bind (Fig. 6.13).

Diagnosis of Tolerance

The diagnosis of tolerance begins by evaluating the clinical history. Tolerance occurs when the drug effect slowly dissipates over weeks or months despite frequent dose increases and this increase in dose does not stabilize (Fig. 6.14). Tolerance is not common; other reasons for dose escalation must therefore be ruled out so appropriate measures can be taken. Also, helpful in the diagnosis of tolerance is a patient diary with documented responses to dose increases over time.

Differential Diagnosis

The differential diagnosis includes true tolerance, delivery system malfunction, or physiologic or psychosocial conditions. Large dose increases

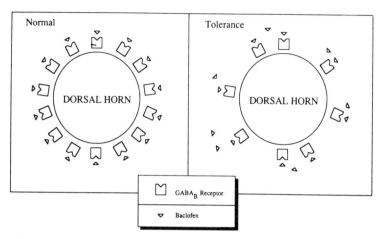

Figure 6.13. Baclofen binds to GABA$_B$ receptors, resulting in reduced spasticity. When baclofen tolerance occurs, it is thought that the number of GABA$_B$ receptors actually decreases. At this time, baclofen is less effective for reducing spasticity since there are fewer GABA$_B$ receptors on which to bind.

over time with no resultant decrease in spasticity should be evaluated. System malfunction, such as a hole or tear in the catheter, may also lead to dose increases with diminished drug effect. If necessary, CSF can be analyzed to verify if the patient is receiving the proper amount of intrathecal baclofen. (Refer to Chapter 8 for assay information and calculation) If inadequate CSF levels are found, this would indicate a system complication, such as a catheter hole. Physiologic or psychosocial conditions may also be responsible for an increase in spasticity. A physiologic condition such as infection or a psychosocial condition of stress typically increases spasticity. Both of these conditions, along with the mechanical system, need to be considered before the patient is diagnosed with tolerance.

Initiating a Drug Holiday

Once the diagnosis of tolerance has been made, a drug holiday may be appropriate. Intrathecal morphine may be considered an appropriate drug to use for a holiday because of its antispastic effect.[51,149,150] Again, morphine is not approved by the FDA for treatment of severe spasticity and its use for this application is considered off-label. Also, intrathecal fentanyl has been reported to be effective for use as an alternative opioid.[112, 151] We have tried bupivacaine, but it has limitations due to lack

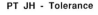

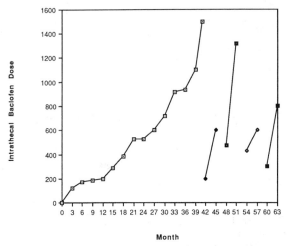

Figure 6.14. A baclofen holiday was implemented for this 43-year-old male with MS after 39 months of receiving the therapy. His dose gradually increased to a maximum of 1500 μg/d. Once this patient was diagnosed with tolerance at month 39, intrathecal morphine was initiated. Owing to side effects from intrathecal morphine and increased spasticity, he was then put back on intrathecal baclofen at a dose of 250 μg/d. Further drug holidays were needed as the dose escalated again. Because of the discomfort this patient experienced while the intrathecal baclofen was decreased prior to beginning another drug holiday, we did not let the dose go higher than 800 μg/d at months 45, 57 and 63.

of availability of high concentrations of the drug, leading to frequent refill. Some clinicians prefer to conduct the drug holiday by gradually withdrawing the patient from intrathecal baclofen and filling the pump reservoir with 0.9% preservative-free normal saline. In these cases, oral antispastic drugs and pain medications are given as substitutes for theduration of the holiday. Because it is more common to use intrathecal morphine for a drug holiday, this application will be discussed.

As with oral baclofen, abruptly withdrawing intrathecal baclofen may lead to serious complications, such as increased spasticity,[57] hypertension,[19,140] autonomic dysreflexia (massive discharge of stimuli from the autonomic nervous system),[19] and seizures.[140,136,137] Intrathecal baclofen must be slowly decreased before beginning intrathecal morphine, and it may be necessary to supplement with oral antispasmodic drugs during this period to provide relief from increasing spasms.

Intrathecal baclofen has been decreased by decrements of 300 to 400 µg every 3 to 4 days in our center without withdrawal effects. In our experience, baclofen can be safely discontinued when the daily rate is approximately 300 to 400 µg. Intrathecal morphine is started at this time.

Starting Intrathecal Morphine

Generally, the initial dose of intrathecal morphine ranges from 0.25 to 0.40 mg/d.[139] In our experience, patients tolerated lower doses of morphine, as many of them developed nausea and vomiting while receiving higher initial doses. The short term side effects of intrathecal morphine include nausea and vomiting, urinary retention, constipation, pruritus, sedation, and possible respiratory depression. Appropriate medication may be used to alleviate or diminish some of these side effects. This may include trimethobenzamide hydrochloride (Tigan) suppositories for nausea, diphenhydramine hydrochloride (Benadryl) for pruritus, and laxatives for constipation. (Refer to Chapter 7 for management of adverse effects associated with intrathecal morphine.) Unfortunately, not every patient receives antispasmodic effects from intrathecal morphine. Furthermore, the drug holiday requires frequent visits for dose adjusting which may create transportation difficulties for some patients. The severity of these side effects may be a reason to terminate the intrathecal morphine drug holiday.

The amount of time a patient remains on intrathecal morphine can vary. For one patient, the holiday lasted only 1 to 2 weeks.[116] For other patients, the average length of the holiday lasted 4 to 8 weeks.[19,128] Typically, patients may continue with intrathecal morphine until they experience intolerable side effects or their spasticity worsens despite morphine dose increases. When these situations occur, intrathecal baclofen is restarted.

Restarting Intrathecal Baclofen

During the absence of intrathecal baclofen, the patient becomes more sensitive to the drug. Physiologically, there are more receptors for intrathecal baclofen to bind to than prior to the drug holiday. Therefore, *the drug must be restarted at a low dose or an overdose may result.* The patient's initial dose at implant, approximately 100 to 300 µg, serves as a general guide for restarting the dose of intrathecal baclofen. Table 6.13 summarizes the interventions required when placing tolerant patients on a "baclofen holiday" and substituting treatment with intrathecal morphine.

Table 6.13. Conducting a Baclofen Holiday and Substituting Treatment with Intrathecal Morphine.

Initiation of a drug holiday

- tapering intrathecal baclofen to prevent withdrawal (typically in increments of 300–400 μg)
- ordering antispasmodics as needed for comfort (such as diazepam, dantrolene sodium, or oral baclofen)

Converting to morphine

- start morphine between 0.25 and 0.40 mg/d (it may be best to start with a lower dose if the patient is not receiving opioids)
- continue for 2–8 weeks (depending on the efficacy and adverse effects associated with intrathecal morphine)

Short-term side effects of intrathecal morphine

- nausea and/or vomiting
- urinary retention
- constipation
- sedation
- pruritus
- possible respiratory changes

Restarting intrathecal baclofen

- restart dose close to original implant dose (typically 100–300 μg/d)
- restarting at a high dose may result in hypotonia or overdose the patient

---

■ CONCLUSION

Chronic, intractable spasticity contributes significantly to the disability of patients with MS or SCI. Severe spasticity often causes pain, interrupts sleep, and interferes with function. While oral antispastic medications and physical therapy are effective for many patients, others do not achieve adequate relief and often experience intolerable side effects. Severe spasticity of spinal origin responds dramatically to the long-term infusion of intrathecal baclofen. The drug can be delivered safely and accurately by a programmable drug pump which permits flexibility with dosing and thus accommodates the individual lifestyle of each patient.

Careful patient selection and screening are required. Refer to Table 6.14 for an abbreviated protocol for screening and initiating treatment. Patients must satisfactorily respond to a trial dose of 100 μg or less. Patients who meet the screening criteria may elect to have the drug pump implanted to facilitate continuous delivery. During the postoperative

Table 6.14. Intrathecal Baclofen for Spinal Spasticity: Protocol (Rush-Presbyterian-St. Luke's Medical Center, Chicago, Ill.)

I. Patient selection

- Patient must have spasticity of spinal origin (MS or SCI).
- Patient mut be unresponsive to oral baclofen and/or experience intolerable side effects.

II. Screening phase

Day 1
- Allow patient to continue taking oral antispastic medications as scheduled.
- Procedure performed in hospital: general ortho-neurosurgery unit.
- Begin with a trial dose of 75μg/lumbar puncture; evaluate for response (drug peaks in approximately 2 h).
- Continuously monitor with portable cardiac/apnea monitor or telemetry with pulse oximetry.
- Record VS prebolus, and 1/2, 1, 2, 4, and 6 h after intrathecal injection of baclofen; evaluate spasticity according to the Ashworth and spasm scores.
- Assess for adverse effects.

Day 2
- If a positive response to 75 μg, implant drug pump.
- If no response to 75μg, repeat the trial with a 100 μg bolus/lumbar puncture.

III. Surgical phase

Day 2 or 3
- Procedure performed with local anesthesia and short-acting intravenous sedatives as needed. (General anesthesia is indicated for patients with severe spasms interfering with positioning.)
- Begin initial baclofen dose at 2× the screening dose that produced an effect.
- Titrate intrathecal baclofen dose every 24 h (postoperatively) until the desired effect is achieved.
- Gradually decrease oral antispastic medications (abrupt withdrawal of baclofen has been associated with hallucinations and seizures).
- Discharge instructions to include information about emerging contacts and procedures.

(Continued)

Table 6.14. (*Continued*)

IV. Long-term management
– Maintain safe and effective therapy.
– Perform refill procedure and adjust dose as necessary (10% to 40% increments).
– Assess for adverse effects and/or system complications.
– Treat overdose with physostigmine: 1–2 mg IV over 5–10 min (adult dose).
– Initiative referrals as necessary.

period, oral antispastic medications are gradually discontinued. The intrathecal dose of baclofen is titrated according to the patient's degree of spasticity and level of function. Adverse effects associated with intrathecal baclofen include drowsiness, weakness in the lower extremities, dizziness, lightheadedness, seizures, headache, and nausea and vomiting.

The primary responsibility of health care professionals participating in long-term care is maintaining safe and effective therapy. Refer to Table 6.15 for typical questions regarding managing patients on intrathecal baclofen. During follow-up visits, spasticity and level of function are evaluated, the pump is refilled with baclofen, and the dose is adjusted as necessary. In addition, the delivery system's performance is evaluated for accuracy. Caution must be taken to avoid accidentally overdosing the patient. Patient education is essential and must be reinforced throughout all phases of the therapy.

Table 6.15. Common Questions Regarding Managing Patients on Intrathecal Baclofen

---

1. Is it safe to mix intrathecal baclofen with intrathecal morphine and administer to patients presenting with pain and spasticity?

There is inadequate experience with the use of intrathecal baclofen in combination with other intrathecal medications to predict efficacy, and the safety of such combination therapy is unknown. It is not recommended that the two drugs be mixed and infused together in the pump because of difficulty performing dose adjustments, unknown stabilty in the pump, and patients potentially becoming tolerant to morphine and requiring dose increases where baclofen increases may no be warranted.

2. Do patients maintained on intrathecal baclofen have a higher incidence of DVTs/PEs?

We have not incurred a higher incidence of DVTs/PEs in patients receiving a chronic infusion of intrathecal baclofen. However, we titrate daily doses to control spasticity and are careful to avoid flaccidity or hypotonia. Unfortunately, patients with MS or SCI are at risk for these complications, and some should be treated prophylactically with coumadin or various filters that trap emboli.

3. When is the best time to initiate rehabilitation services — immediately after the pump is implanted and spasticity is reduced, or several weeks after implant, when the intrathecal dose has stabilized?

There are arguments that support either time period. Depending on the patient and his/her expected outcome, rehabilitation may be initiated as soon as proper healing has occurred and spasticity is reduced. It may require several weeks to precisely adjust the patients dose, particularly for patients who ambulate, and delaying rehabilitation for a short period of time may be warranted to optimize muscle tone.

4. How does intrathecal baclofen affect a patient with a history of autonomic dysreflexia?

Although abrupt withdrawal of intrathecal baclofen may cause an autonomic dysreflexic episode, a continuous infusion does not potentiate or exacerbate this condition. Other sources of nociceptive stimuli are known to "trigger" autonomic dysreflexic episodes.

7

Intraspinal Morphine for Pain

Pain is an enormous social and economic problem. The treatment of chronic pain is also controversial, in part because of the subjectivity of the complaint. Most health care professionals have been trained to treat acute pain, expecting to see changes in vital signs, facial grimacing, and guarding behavior. However, in the chronic pain patient these signs are not evident. Therefore, the only reliable indicator of the presence of pain is the patient's self-report. This may prove challenging to the health professional when assessing pain in the patient who reports a pain intensity of 10 on a 0 to 10 scale but does not "look as if he/she is in pain." Reports of intensity scores that do not correlate with behavior are common and may also reflect coping strategies and other patient-specific variables.

Pain affects all parts of the patient's life. The International Association for the Study of Pain addresses the multifactorial nature of pain: "Pain is an unpleasant sensory and emotional experience, associated with actual or potential damage, or described in such terms."[152] Thus, pain is more than an action potential in the nervous system. Pain has enormous emotional, financial, and social consequences not only for the patient, but also for the patient's support persons.

Because pain is multifactorial, the treatment of chronic pain must include many options and be delivered by numerous disciplines working together with the patient. In both malignant and nonmalignant pain, interventions designed to treat the cause of the pain should be instituted. This may include the use of chemotherapy or radiation therapy in the cancer patient, or surgery, if appropriate, in the nonmalignant pain patient.[153]

When the source of the pain cannot be directly treated, pain management techniques include nonpharmacologic and pharmacologic interventions. Nonpharmacologic interventions include physical therapies directed at recovering or improving muscle function, and psychological techniques, such as relaxation, guided imagery, distraction, and hypnosis. The many pharmacologic treatment options available include nonopioids (including nonsteroidal antiinflammatory drugs and acetaminophen), opioids, and adjunct drugs (such as anticonvulsants, antidepressants, corticosteroids, and others). The vast majority of patients can obtain good relief from oral medications in combination with nonpharmacologic interventions (Table 7.1). When oral medications delivered by these methods are ineffective, or when side effects occur, alternative delivery methods may be considered, such as intraspinal drugs administered via implanted pumps (Fig. 7.1).

To understand the reason for the use of intraspinal drugs delivered via implanted pumps for pain, one must first understand pain physiology.

■ PHYSIOLOGY OF PAIN

Understanding the rationale for spinal drug delivery requires knowledge of the physiology of pain transmission. Pain is initiated by some type of thermal, chemical, or mechanical stimulus. These may include burns, exposure to acidic or alkaline substances, or trauma. These stimuli lead to the generation of an action potential in primary sensory neurons—also called nociceptors. The pain message is transmitted along these neurons as they course through the periphery and enter into the spinal cord. These fibers synapse in the dorsal horn of the spinal cord with neurons that ascend to higher centers in the CNS.

It is this synaptic site within the dorsal horn of the spinal cord that is key to understanding the use of opioids to relieve pain, as well as other potential analgesics currently under study. The primary sensory neurons

Table 7.1. Interventions to relieve pain.

Pharmacologic	Nonpharmacologic
Nonopioids	Cognitive-behavioral therapies
NSAIDS	Distraction
Acetaminophen	Guided imagery
Opioids	Relaxation
Adjuvant drugs	Hypnosis
Antidepressants	Ablative prcedures
Anticonvulsants	Nerve blocks
Corticosteroids	Neurosurgical procedures
Local anesthetics	
Others	

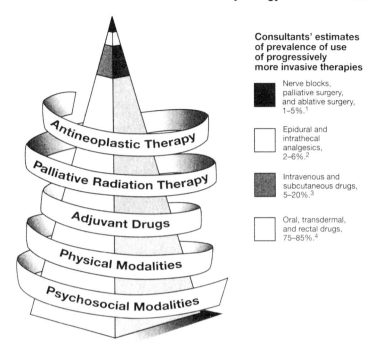

Consultants' estimates
of prevalence of use
of progressively
more invasive therapies

Nerve blocks,
palliative surgery,
and ablative surgery,
1–5%.[1]

Epidural and
intrathecal
analgesics,
2–6%.[2]

Intravenous and
subcutaneous drugs,
5–20%.[3]

Oral, transdermal,
and rectal drugs,
75–85%.[4]

Figure 7.1. Pain management strategies: a hierarchy. Many pharmacologic and nonpharmacologic therapies are available in the treatment of pain. The pyramid illustrates that least invasive methods may be effective in the majority of cancer patients, while invasive procedures are indicated in fewer patients. Although developed to illustrate cancer pain management, this hierarchy may also demonstrate the care of nonmalignant pain. (Reprinted from Jacox et al.[153])

release neurotransmitters such as substance P, vasoactive intestinal polypeptide (VIP), cholecystokinin (CCK), calcitonin gene-related peptide (CGRP), excitatory amino acids, and other substances. These substances bind to receptors on ascending neurons and, if existing in sufficient quantities, cause the generation of an action potential in these neurons. The pain message is then transmitted to higher centers, where it is believed the individual actually perceives pain (Fig. 7.2).

One theoretical approach to the inhibition of pain is the administration of drugs to block the release of these neurotransmitters. By blocking the release of neurotransmitters in the spinal cord, pain transmission would be blocked before the message reaches the level of perception. In fact,

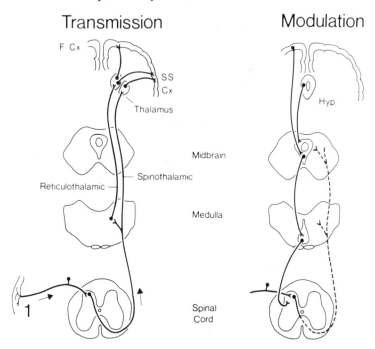

Figure 7.2. The pathophysiology of pain. Pain is transmitted through peripheral sensory fibers that synapse in the spinal cord with ascending tracts of neurons. These tracts transmit pain to higher centers of the CNS, where it is believed the individual becomes aware of the existence of pain. (Reprinted with permission from Fields.[154])

when opioids are administered systemically or intraspinally, they bind to opioid receptors presynaptically on the primary afferent neurons. When adequate binding occurs, neurotransmitter release is inhibited. This effect inhibits further transmission of the pain message.

The rationale for administering opioids intraspinally is that delivery of drugs directly to their site of action would allow the use of lower doses of drug, potentially leading to fewer side effects. Most patients receiving intrathecal morphine or other opioids experience fewer episodes of sedation and less constipation than patients taking systemic opioids. Unfortunately, nausea and vomiting are common in the initial infusion period, although they rarely persist for periods beyond 24 to 48 hours.

■ PATIENT SELECTION

Intractable Pain

The criteria for choosing intrathecal opioid therapy for pain include the presence of intractable pain or the development of severe, unmanageable side effects with systemic opioid therapy (Table 7.2). "Intractable" pain is that which has not been controlled despite aggressive use of systemic opioids and adjuvant drugs, such as antidepressants, anticonvulsants, and other agents. Patients often present with "intractable" pain when they have not been given a strong opioid, have been given inappropriately low doses of opioids, or have not been given adjuvant drugs.

Several reports suggest that patients who are receiving high-dose systemic opioids without adequate relief are unlikely to obtain significant pain relief with intraspinal opioids.[155] When evaluating these patients for pump implantation the clinician must be prepared to consider alternative drugs if spinal opioids fail, including local anesthetics or other agents.

Adverse Effects to Systemic Opioids

Side effects to oral opioids must be aggressively and appropriately treated prior to being considered unmanageable. Many patients experience nausea and vomiting with systemic opioid therapy. Treatment with antiemetics for the first 24 to 48 hours or switching to an alternative opioid usually relieves these effects. Sedation generally diminishes after the first 24 to 48 hours. When sedation persists, oral caffeine or psychostimulants, such as methylphenidate, can be given. Antihistamines can be used to treat pruritus, which also subsides after 1 or 2 days in most patients. Urinary retention may occur with systemic opioids; this effect may also occur with spinal opioids. Patients with severe respiratory disease, such as congestive obstructive pulmonary disease or emphysema, may be extremely sensitive to the respiratory depressant effects of

Table 7.2. Selection criteria.

Intractable pain
Unmanageable side effects with oral opioids
Location of pain below midcervical dermatome
Adequate caregiver support
Willingness to participate in rehabilitation
Psychological screening yields appropriate findings

systemic opioids. Alternative systemic opioids should be tried when any of these side effects persist. Case studies indicate that patients may try several different opioids before finding one that leads to fewer adverse effects. When these efforts fail, patients are considered appropriate candidates for implanted pumps for pain.

Location of the Pain

The location of the pain must also be considered when evaluating potential patients. Pain originating from nerve roots below the level of the cervical spine is generally accepted as appropriate for intraspinal therapy, although at least one report indicates that intraspinal opioid treatment for head and neck cancer can be successful.[27] Patients with metastatic tumors that cause cord compression at the lumbar or low thoracic level may not be candidates since the tumor could obstruct catheter placement or drug flow.

Psychosocial Factors

Patient resources and caregiver support are essential when considering potential candidates for intraspinal therapy. The patient must be able to return to the outpatient center for suture removal, pump refill, and dose modification. Many home care agencies now have the skill to refill implanted pumps, and some have the equipment to allow reprogramming of pumps. The use of home care agencies varies by clinician. Some routinely consult home care agencies for all maintenance, whereas others limit referral to home care only when patients are too disabled to leave the home. These factors should be examined early since home health services may not be available in all locations and all third-party payers may not reimburse for these services.

Nonmalignant pain patients must also agree to participate in rehabilitation after pump implantation. This may include behavior modification to stop smoking or lose weight, physical therapy, exercise, vocational counseling or psychological support. Psychological screening prior to pump implantation helps clinicians determine whether the patient is able to participate fully in the pain program. This diagnostic workup, which may include the Minnesota Multiphasic Personality Index (MMPI), the Multidimensional Pain Index (MPI), the Beck Depression Index, and the McGill Pain Questionnaire, helps identify psychological difficulties that may require treatment prior to pump therapy. The psychologist may also determine procedures that will help augment spinal therapy, including cognitive-behavioral techniques such as relaxation, guided imagery, hypnosis, and others.

Screening

A trial of opioids is necessary prior to the placement of an expensive implanted device; however, the type of screening used varies widely. The most frequently used drug trials include (1) an epidural bolus dose of morphine; (2) repeated intermittent doses of epidural morphine administered through a temporary catheter over a 24- to 48-hour period; (3) a continuous epidural infusion over a 2- to 3-day period; or (4) a one-time intrathecal bolus (Table 7.3). Another, less common screening technique is the continuous intrathecal infusion of drug via an external catheter; however, the risk of infection makes this approach less acceptable.

Continuous epidural infusions most closely emulate the final therapy and allow the clinician to interact with the patient over a prolonged time. Patients are allowed to take supplemental oral opioids during the trial, and activity is monitored. Apnea monitors or pulse oximeters are used in some settings to evaluate respiratory effects of the opioid. Criteria used to evaluate efficacy during the trial include reduction in pain intensity, increase in function (if reasonable given the patient's disease), and decrease in supplemental opioid use. Occasionally, patients with nonmalignant pain may take very high doses of supplemental opioids during screening with the epidural infusion, or may not engage in any activity. These are potential indicators of a poor prognosis, since these patients are not actively participating in the therapy. Unfortunately, this type of screening procedure prolongs hospitalization, increases cost, and may not be reimbursed.

Bolus administration requires a shorter screening period, but side effects may be more pronounced. Patients also state after implantation that the degree of pain relief is never so intense as that obtained during bolus screening, even when comparable or larger doses are used. The reason for this phenomenon is unclear; it may be due to high peak levels of drug. One uncontrolled study suggests that trial periods using epidural bolus doses are not predictive of initial dose requirements of intrathecal drug, but are effective in predicting patient side effects.[169]

The drug that will be used during long-term therapy should be the agent used during the screening trial. Morphine is currently the most commonly used intrathecal agent, but some clinicians may choose to use alternative agents. If these agents are being considered, they should be included in the screening to evaluate efficacy and adverse effects. Some investigators use placebo as part of their screening protocol, purportedly to rule out those patients with psychogenic pain. When given a placebo for pain relief, a large percentage of the population will respond.[170] Therefore, the addition of a saline control does not effectively rule out patients with psychological difficulties. Furthermore, for ethical reasons,

Table 7.3. Intraspinal drug therapy for pain: screening techniques.

Author	Screening method (with doses if indicated)	No. pts	Type of pts	Screening criteria	Final therapy	Outcome criteria
Anderson[27]	Continuous epidural	9	Head and neck cancer	VAS,* side effects	SynchroMed, IT (dose 10% of epidural trial)	VAS
Auld[156]	Epidural bolus 1 mg MSO$_4$ and 2 mL saline	43	Nonmalignant pain	Good to excellent relief	Infusaid, epidural	Not defined
Brazenor[157]	None	25	Malignant (23) Nonmalignant (3)	None cited	Infusaid	Functional capacity; quality of analgesia (excellent, good); other analgesics
Coombs[158–160]	Bolus epidural (0.06–0.08 mg/kg)	7 (1982) 10 (1983) 14 (1984)	Cancer (6) and nonmalignant (1) Cancer (9) and nonmalignant (1) Cancer	50% reduction in VAS for at least 8 h	Infusaid	McGill, VAS, oral opioid use, Zung Self Rating Depression Scale

Follett[161]	Bolus intrathecal (1–4 mg; based on 1/10 oral dose)	37	Cancer (35) Nonmalignant (2)	50% reduction in NRS[†] for 12–16 h (if fail, double dose and repeat)	Infusaid, SynchroMed	
Hassenbusch[162]	Continuous epidural 2–4 days	41	Cancer pain	30% reduction in VAS or NRS; epidural dose ↓ 30 mg/day (41/69 [5.4%] met criteria)	Infusaid, epidural	VAS, NRS; oral dose
Krames[163]	Bolus intrathecal (1.0–2.5 mg MSO$_4$ then bolus epidural (5–10 mg MSO$_4$ × days)	17	Cancer (16) Nonmalignant pain (1)	VAS–50% reduction	Infusaid	Pain relief 0–5[‡] 5, no pain; 4, mild pain, infrequent nonnarcotics; 3, moderate pain, frequent nonnarcotics; 2, moderate pain, infrequent narcotics; 1, moderate pain, frequent narcotics; 0, poor pain relief, frequent narcotics.

Table 7.3. (*Continued*)

Author	Screening method (with doses if indicated)	No. pts	Type of pts	Screening criteria	Final therapy	Outcome criteria
Onofrio[28,164]	Bolus intrathecal (0.75–2 mg MSO_4)	53	Cancer	"Fair response" for at least 6 h	Infusaid	Mobility (1, 2, 3); supplemental opiates
Penn[165, 166]	Continuous epidural (4.8–14.4 mg) 2–3 days	14 43	Cancer Cancer (35) Nonmalignant (8)	NRS–50% reduction; supplemental opioids–50% reduction	Infusaid SynchroMed	Excellent: Pain 0–3; 50% ↓ oral supplements; increased ADL Good: Pain 4–6; <50% ↓ oral supplements; increased ADL Poor: Pain 7–10; no change in supplements; no change in ADL
Shetter[167]	Bolus epidural 3.75 mg–7.5 mg q 12° × 2–6 days	24	Cancer	Subjective evaluate; supplemental opioids	Ommaya, Infusaid	E, Excellent. Postoperative pain reduction > 75%. Supplemental narcotics usage < 3.5 parenteral morphine equivalents per day. No further treatment for pain.

| Waterman[168] | Bolus epidural 0.5% bupivacaine; 3 mg MSO$_4$ than continuous epidural | 33 | Cancer | Not cited | Infusaid, Port-A-Cath, epidural catheter | G, Good. Pain reduction > 50%. Supplemental narcotics required but no further treatment for pain.
P, Poor. Pain reduction < 25%. Supplemental narcotics required, and further hospitalization or treatment need for pain control.
Not cited |

patients should be informed that they might be given a placebo during the trial.

How well screening trials predict the efficacy of intrathecal opioids delivered via implanted pump is unclear, since this question has not been prospectively studied. In a recent retrospective, multicenter review of 429 patients, screening method was not related to improved outcome, including greater pain relief or increased activities of daily living.[171] As a result of the lack of systematic study, clinicians must use their best judgement when choosing the appropriate screening technique, taking into consideration the physical health of the patient, the drugs to be used during therapy, and cost factors.

■ INTRATHECAL DRUG DOSING

Postoperative Period

Medications may be injected into the implanted pump during surgery and infused immediately, with titration usually beginning on the first or second postoperative day. Equianalgesic dosing between systemic, epidural, and intrathecal drug administration has not been firmly established, making the determination of an effective starting dose difficult. The dose of morphine effective during epidural screening may not predict the dose needed via the pump. One uncontrolled study indicated that the epidural morphine dose did not predict later intrathecal doses, but rather served as a guide to possible side effects.[169]

Using bolus administration, Nordberg determined that after intramuscular, epidural, and intrathecal injections of morphine, the conversion from the epidural to the intrathecal route appears to be 24:1 (Fig. 7.3).[172] This study also suggests that the relative potencies of IV to epidural to intrathecal morphine are 1:2:20–40. However, because this study was based on bolus administration, this ratio is probably not accurate for continuous delivery in people with chronic pain. Based on extensive clinical experience, Krames recommended a 10:1 conversion, so that 10 mg of epidural morphine is approximately equal to 1 mg of intrathecal morphine.[22] Even less information is available regarding conversion of systemic opioids to intrathecal doses. Thus, because starting doses are difficult to predict, frequent titration is necessary.

Long-term Management

Decisions regarding dose changes are based on the patient's report of pain intensity and the presence of any side effects. While the patient is

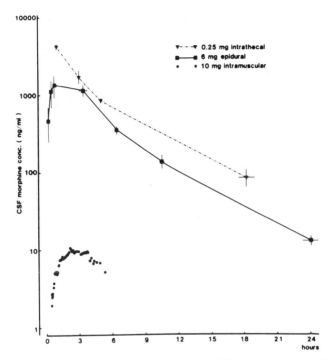

Figure 7.3. Levels of morphine within the CSF after intramuscular, epidural, and intrathecal injections. (Reprinted with permission from Nordberg.[172])

hospitalized, the dose is increased approximately 10 to 25% each day or twice daily after surgery. These escalations continue less frequently after discharge. After hospitalization, the dose is increased based on patient reports of pain intensity, activity level, and supplemental opioid use. It is not uncommon to see patients well controlled in the hospital but requiring significant increases in dose during the first 1 to 2 months. This reflects a return to previous levels of activity and to rehabilitation.

The dose of intrathecal morphine needed to control pain is highly variable, similar to the variability seen with systemic opioids. Yaksh and Onofrio retrospectively surveyed 19 physicians regarding chronic morphine doses administered intrathecally via implanted pumps.[173] The mean daily dose of morphine was 4.8 mg at week 1, mg, 16 mg at approximately 6 months, and 21 mg at 1 year. The dose at 1 year reflected a small number of patients (N = 10), and there was great variability in doses at each time frame.

In a recent retrospective study of 429 patients receiving intraspinal morphine delivered by implanted, programmable pumps, the doses varied based on the patients' diagnosis and the type of pain experienced. For example, for the 128 cancer patients receiving intrathecal opioids by an implanted pump, the mean intrathecal dose at 1 week was 7.7 mg/d, at 6 months 14.2 mg/d, and at 12 months 14.2 mg/d.[171] This is in contrast to the 264 nonmalignant-pain patients, whose dose was increased in a linear fashion, from 3.2 mg/d, to 5.5 mg/d, and 7.8 mg/d at 1 week, 6 months and 12 months, respectively (Fig. 7.4). Additionally, patients with neuropathic pain required statistically significant increases in dose when compared to patients who did not have this type of pain. These differences in dose between cancer and nonmalignant-pain patients may represent greater clinician comfort with escalating doses in cancer patients, or the need for higher doses in cancer patients due to more intense pain stimuli or previous exposure to systemic opioids. The need for higher doses in patients with neuropathic pain is also consistent with reports of reduced efficacy of systemic opioids in relieving neuropathic pain.

Intrathecal Morphine Doses Delivered by Implanted Drug Pump

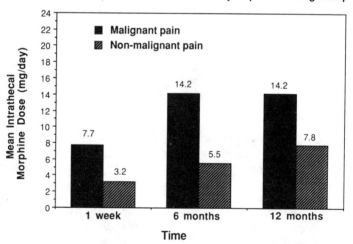

Figure 7.4. In a retrospective study of 429 patients, 128 patients were diagnosed with cancer and 264 patients had nonmalignant pain. The mean intrathecal morphine doses for these two groups increased from 1 week, 6 months, and 12 months. The mean doses for the cancer pain group tended to plateau at from 6 to 12 months, while mean doses for the nonmalignant pain group started lower and rose gradually in a linear fashion.[171]

Sudden onset of pain or rapidly escalating doses after a period of stable dosing suggests either system-related complications or the development of a new physiologic problem. Delivery system-related problems, described in Chapter 8, are usually associated with the catheter and may include dislodgment, cracking or kinking. The patient must also be immediately evaluated for potential disease recurrence or the onset of new painful syndromes. For example, complaints of back pain in a patient with lung cancer who previously described thoracic pain, may herald the presence of spinal metastases. Because of the risk of cord compression, this patient should be seen immediately by the oncologist.

When patients complain of little relief with intraspinal opioids, and system malfunction has been ruled out, alternative agents are necessary. Our first choice would be the use of another opioid, such as hydromorphone (Dilaudid). Available in a 10 mg/mL concentration, 1 mg hydromorphone is generally considered to be approximately equal to 5 mg morphine. Patients who do not obtain relief, or who develop side effects from morphine, may benefit from hydromorphone. This agent is a good alternative when high concentrations of drug are needed, since using the 1:5 conversion indicates that the 10 mg/mL concentration of hydromorphone is approximately to 50 mg/mL of morphine.

The next most commonly used class of agents, particularly in the relief of neuropathic pain, is the local anesthetics. These agents are typically added to the opioid and delivered in doses starting at 1.25 to 2.5 mg/d. Doses as high as 100 mg/d have been reported with the use of external intrathecal catheters and pumps in cancer patients[175]; however, these extreme doses can produce significant sensorimotor weakness, can lead to hypotension due to sympathetic blockade, and would require extremely high flow rates using implanted pumps. The most frequently used agent, bupivicaine, is available in 0.25% and 0.75% preservative-free solutions.

Because of the use of two drugs within the implanted pump, dose titration requires extreme care. As the dose of the local anesthetic is increased, so is the dose of the opioid, which may lead to significant adverse effects such as respiratory depression. Patients may require increases in each drug separately. For example, the patient who is sedated but continuing to experience pain may require an increase in local anesthetic dose but not an increase in the dose of the opioid. Conversely, patients with reduced sensory perception in the lower extremities but with continued pain may require an increase in opioids but not an increase in the local anesthetic.

When these efforts fail, other agents described in Chapter 5 that have been found to be analgesic when administered intrathecally may be used. However, the clinician must be aware that the use of drugs for pain other than morphine constitutes off-label use of the drug pumps. Although this is a common phenomenon in clinical practice (for example, antidepressants are indicated for the effect on depression but are frequently used to treat pain), the physician must carefully weigh the advantages of using these drugs against possible legal concerns and reimbursement issues.

Tolerance

The frequency and mechanism of analgesic tolerance to spinal opioids are unclear and somewhat controversial. This effect was documented early in the use of intraspinal morphine,[176] but other investigators contend that increases in dose are uncommon,[175] reflect advancing disease,[22,175] are due to delivery system complications[156] or may be associated with neuropathic pain.[155] In a retrospective, multiphysician study of 163 patients, almost half of patients had less than a two-fold increase in the dose by 3 months.[173]

In our experience, significant dose increases occur in the initial 3-month postimplant period. Rather than reflecting tolerance, this increase represents dose finding. The majority of patients, then, have doses that plateau for long periods of time, often for years. Continued need for increases is often associated with catheter dislodgment or neuropathic pain. Evaluation of the delivery system is necessary to rule out complications. Conversion to a different agent may provide relief if the system is intact.

Several centers routinely use "drug holidays" to reduce the need for increasing doses of drug. Two theories underlie the rationale for a drug holiday. Physiologically, receptors will be cleared of the drug once it is discontinued, thereby leading to the need for less drug once the drug is reintroduced. Psychologically, some clinicians contend that nonmalignant pain patients should be periodically "reminded" of their pain, so that they will appreciate the amount of relief they are receiving from the intraspinal agent. In our experience, the holiday is a painful period that requires expert management to prevent and treat potentially dangerous withdrawal effects (Table 7.4). Additionally, although the initial dose requirement is reduced when intrathecal opioids are restarted, these doses often require rapid increases to amounts near or at previous levels.

Thus, the way to manage analgesic tolerance remains unclear. Improved catheter systems will potentially reduce the complications that mimic tolerance. The availability of alternative agents to treat neuropathic pain more effectively will improve the overall efficacy of intraspinal drug delivery. Finally, large multicenter, prospective trials will allow clear determination of the frequency of tolerance and factors that may lead to its occurrence.

Table 7.4. Symptoms of withdrawal from systemic opioids.

Yawning
Agitation
Sleeplessness
Rhinorrhea
Abdominal cramping
Diarrhea
Piloerection
Diaphoresis
Dilated pupils
Nausea and vomiting
Lacrimation
Anorexia
Muscle spasms
Low back pain
Seizures (if previously taking meperidine)

■ SUPPLEMENTAL OPIOIDS

Postoperative Period

During the immediate postoperative period, patients will require supplemental opioids to manage the pain associated with the incisions and the mass of the pump in the subcutaneous pocket. Patients previously receiving opioids will require higher doses of drug than might patients who did not tolerate systemic morphine. Unless the patient is NPO or the oral route is contraindicated, supplemental opioids should be given orally. If unable to tolerate oral administration, alternative routes include rectal, sublingual, buccal, or intravenous delivery. Most patients require supplemental opioids for incisional pain for 3 to 7 days after surgery. Wearing loose clothing around the waist and holding a pillow or folded towel against the pump incision during coughing or ambulation help alleviate incisional pain.

Long-Term Management

Many patients who have been taking systemic opioids regularly prior to pump implantation now require reduced dosages. Gradually reduce these supplemental opioids by approximately 25% to 50% each day to prevent withdrawal phenomenon. Withdrawal, or the abstinence syndrome, occurs even in the face of intraspinal drug delivery because, although more drug reaches receptors in the spinal cord, less drug is available to bind to opiate receptors systemically. This phenomenon (described in Table 7.4) is a result of the pharmacologic activity of opioids and does not reflect psychological dependence or other emotional problems.

The additional use of supplemental opioids in cancer patients is essential. Patients should have ready access to short-acting opioids, such as immediate-release morphine, to treat periods of incident or break-through pain. Continuous need for supplemental drug may indicate an inadequate intrathecal dose and should warrant upward increases.

The chronic use of supplemental opioids in nonmalignant-pain patients is considered controversial by some professionals who treat patients with pain. Some fear regulatory scrutiny and retribution. Other professionals are concerned about the potential for tolerance and long-term side effects. There is also fear that oral opioids are a temporary solution to a long-term problem and that patients must come to accept their chronic pain and actively pursue nondrug therapies and rehabilitation measures.

Other pain experts have successfully administered chronic opioid therapy, alone or in conjunction with intraspinal opioids, without adverse events. They argue that these medications allow patients to lead productive lives and participate in rehabilitation more effectively. Patients are given clear instructions regarding the use of these medications (Table 7.5). Limits are set to help patients learn the skills necessary to regulate their own medications.

Other Supplemental Medications

Many other medications are useful in the management of chronic pain. Nonopioids, such as the nonsteroidal antiinflammatory drugs (NSAIDs) and acetaminophen, block prostaglandin synthesis and are especially effective in reducing bone and joint pain. Tricyclic antidepressants act by blocking reuptake of norepinephrine and serotonin and are particularly useful in relieving neuropathic pain. Additionally, these agents may cause sedation, and thus, if taken before bedtime, assist sleep. Their mood-elevating effect is also advantageous in chronic-pain patients, who are often depressed. There is evidence that the newer, serotonin-selective antidepressant agents may not be as effective in relieving pain. Anticonvulsants are effective in alleviating neuropathic pain by blocking ion channels. Other drug and nondrug therapies can be useful in treating chronic pain. Resources for health professionals and patients interested in pain are listed in the appendices.

Table 7.5. Patient education regarding supplemental
medicines for nonmalignant pain.

You are receiving a set amount of medicine delivered by the
pump into the area around the spine each day.

Medicine _____

Daily dose _____

Some patients never need additional medicine. Others have
periods of increased pain associated with activity or weather. Still
others have a type of pain that is not managed well by the
medicine in the pump, and they always have some level of pain.
For these reasons, we may order additional medicines to work with
the medicine given by the pump.

Many different types of medicine are available. For example,
nonopioids such as aspirin, acetaminophen (Tylenol), or ibuprofen
(Motrin) help relieve bone or joint pain, such as arthritis.
Antidepressants relieve burning, tingling, and electrical pain. They
also help sleep and improve mood. Anticonvulsants (antiseizure
medicine) may help burning and tingling pain. Opioids (narcotics)
may be needed to treat certain types of pain.

Your medications:

Drug _____ Dose _____ When and how often you should take

_____
_____
_____
_____

We will provide prescriptions for these medications at each refill.
If you have a bad pain day, you may take:

_____
_____

Keep in mind that the prescription must last until your next
refill. We will not order more medicine between visits. If you take
more medicine one day, you must use less a day or 2 later. This
allows you the freedom to regulate your own medicine. These are
important skills to help you learn to manage chronic pain.

Some patients find it helpful to divide the pills that they can
regulate into weekly bottles. This helps you control the amount
you take so that you have enough medicine to last until the next
refill. Others find that keeping a diary is helpful, adding up how
many pills they use each day. Try nondrug therapy to help with
increased periods of pain, including heat or cold, massage,
vibration, and relaxation techniques.

Other instructions: _____

■ ADVERSE INTRASPINAL DRUG EFFECTS

Immediate Effects

Immediate adverse effects have been noted with intraspinal opioid therapy (Table 7.6), particularly when patients have not been treated with systemic opioids prior to therapy. Nausea and vomiting are common, generally last 24 to 48 hours, and are easily treated with antiemetics. If nausea or vomiting persists and other causes have been ruled out, switch to an alternative opioid. Implanted pumps have been approved by the FDA for the use of morphine; however, numerous investigators have successfully administered hydromorphone and other agents.

Urinary retention is more common in males with benign prostatic hypertrophy or patients who have had previous genitourinary surgery. Intermittent catheterization may be necessary in the initial 24 to 48 hours; however, in our experience no patient has required long-term bladder catheterization.

Pruritus may also occur, especially over the face, cheeks, and nose. Although the mechanism of pruritus is unknown, diphenhydramine, administered orally or intermuscularly, is useful in alleviating this side effect. Only one patient in our care continues to complain of mild itching. However, she has a long history of dermatologic complaints, including frequent rashes, and treats the itching successfully with moisturizers.

Respiratory depression is a feared consequence of intraspinal opioid administration. Fortunately, this effect is rare, particularly in patients

Table 7.6. Reported side effects of intrathecal morphine.

Immediate	Delayed
Nausea and vomiting	Diminished libido
Urinary retention	Infertility/amenorrhea
Pruritus	Constipation
Respiratory depression	Myoclonus
	Edema
	Facial flushing
	Arthralgias
	Nail bed discoloration
	Diaphoresis

previously exposed to opioids. In a meta-analysis of data representing 16 centers, severe respiratory depression occurred in only 0.6% of patients.[34] Monitoring with apnea monitors or pulse oximetry in the initial period provides early assessment. When it does appear, respiratory depression is usually due to errors during the refilling procedure. Other iatrogenic causes must be carefully avoided including mistakes in drug delivery (e.g., injection of drug into the side port when intending to access the reservoir or inadvertently injecting into the subcutaneous space) programming errors, too rapid dose escalation, or excessive bolus doses.

Naloxone can be used to treat respiratory depression but should be used with caution in patients receiving opioids. Naloxone, an opioid antagonist, preferentially binds to opioid receptors. When given to a patient who has been receiving systemic or intraspinal opioids, naloxone will reverse the effects, side effects as well as analgesic effects, and will precipitate the withdrawal phenomenon. An algorithm for the emergency treatment of intrathecal morphine overdose is included in Table 7.7.

Delayed Effects

Long-term effects are now becoming apparent as larger numbers of patients receive intraspinal opioids for extended time periods. Males report decreased libido and difficulty with achieving or maintaining an erection while receiving intrathecal opioids,[177] which is successfully treated with intramuscular testosterone 100 to 200 mg every 3 or 4 weeks. A patch impregnated with testosterone is now available for transdermal delivery (Testoderm Transdermal System; Alza). Females often describe amenorrhea within 1 or 2 months after beginning intrathecal opioid therapy, and the effect on libido in females may be similar to that seen in males. This effect of spinal opioids on sexuality and fertility requires further study.

Constipation has been noted with intraspinal morphine, although there are no studies that compare the degree and mechanism of constipation occurring with spinal opioids to systemic opioid administration. Stool softeners and laxatives may be necessary to relieve constipation.

Myoclonus is an adverse effect noted with both epidural and intrathecal administration, as well as with intravenous infusions. Although myoclonus appears to be dose related, some patients develop myoclonic jerks at relatively low doses. Reducing the intraspinal opioid dose or changing to an alternative opioid may provide relief. Oral baclofen (an antispasmodic), clonazepam, or a benzodiazepine may also be necessary to relieve the very uncomfortable myoclonic jerks. In severe cases the opioid may be discontinued.

Table 7.7. Emergency procedure for morphine intrathecal/epidural overdose.

SynchroMed infusion system
  Programmable drug pump implanted in abdominal wall connected to an intrathecal or epidural catheter. Implanted pump contains an 18-mL drug reservoir and may have more than one port (a drug reservoir port and a catheter access port; see reverse side).

Symptoms
  Respiratory depression with or without concomitant CNS depression (i.e., dizziness, sedation, euphoria, anxiety), seizures, respiratory arrest.*

Actions

```
┌─────────────────────────────────────────────┐
│  Maintain airway/breathing/circulation.     │
│  Respiratory resuscitation and intubation   │
│  may be necessary.                          │
└─────────────────────────────────────────────┘
                       ↓
       ┌─────────────────────────────────┐
       │  Give naloxone (Narcan) 0.4–2 mg │
       │  intravenously.*†                │
       └─────────────────────────────────┘
                       ↓
   ┌─────────────────────────────────────────────┐
   │  If not contraindicated, withdraw 30–40 mL of│
   │  CSF through the catheter access port or by  │
   │  lumbar puncture to reduce CSF morphine      │
   │  concentration.                              │
   └─────────────────────────────────────────────┘
                       ↓
     ┌───────────────────────────────────────┐
     │  Empty pump reservoir to stop drug     │
     │  flow (see reverse side). Record amount│
     │  withdrawn.                            │
     └───────────────────────────────────────┘
```

Response   ↓   No response

    ↓   ↓

┌────────────────────────────────────┐ ┌──────────────────────┐
│ Continue to monitor closely for   │ │ Continue to perform │
│ symptom recurrence. Since the   │ │ life-sustaining   │
│ duration of IV Narcan's effects is │ │ measures.   │
│ shorter than intrathecal/epidural │ └──────────────────────┘
│ morphine, repeated administration │
│ may be necessary.*   │
└────────────────────────────────────┘

  ↓   ↓
No   Recurrence
recurrence   ↓

```
┌─────────────────────────────────────────────────────────┐
│ Repeat Narcan every 2–3 min to maintain adequate        │
│ respiration.*† For continuous IV infusion see Narcan    │
│ package insert.†                                         │
└─────────────────────────────────────────────────────────┘
                          ↓
┌─────────────────────────────────────────────────────────┐
│ If no response is observed after 10 mg Narcan, the      │
│ diagnosis of narcotic-induced toxicity should be        │
│ questioned.*†                                           │
└─────────────────────────────────────────────────────────┘
                          ↓
┌─────────────────────────────────────────────────────────┐
│ Call physician: _____ │
│ Telephone:  (      ) _____  │
└─────────────────────────────────────────────────────────┘
```

*Infumorph (preservative-free morphine sulfate sterile solution) manufacturer's package insert (Wyeth-Ayerst).
†Narcan (naloxone hydrochloride) manufacturer's package insert (DuPont).
NOTE: Drug information is also found in the Physician's Desk Reference (PDR).

Other unusual long-term effects have been described. Dependent edema can be significant. We have seen extreme cases that led to venous stasis ulcers and skin infections. Oral antidiuretics and elevation of the affected extremities will provide only partial resolution. Facial flushing and diaphoresis have also been reported. Arthralgias affecting multiple joints can occur after opioid administration, and have been described in patients receiving spinal opioids. Several clinicians have seen fingernails change color to a dark brown, similar to the color changes described after systemic 5-fluorouracil (a chemotherapeutic agent). The mechanisms for these effects are unknown, and further investigation is necessary.

■ PATIENT EDUCATION

Patient and family education is essential and should begin during the first meeting. An informed patient is more able to participate in the treatment plan, is more compliant, and has more realistic expectations about the therapy. This ultimately improves outcome. Another rationale for thorough patient education is ethicolegal, to assure that the informed consent is truly based on patient understanding.

Patient education prior to pump implantation should include an explanation for the rationale for intraspinal opioid therapy for pain; information about the screening; information on perioperative, postoperative, and long-term care; and details regarding the device. Risks and benefits must be specifically addressed, and patients should be aware of the potential costs of therapy. Patients often express anxiety regarding the operative procedure, especially if they will remain conscious during surgery. They also need to understand the tools used to assess pain so they may more actively participate in their care. Sample pain intensity measures appear in Table 7.8.

Family members and caregivers must be included in the teaching plan, and written material should be provided to supplement verbal instruction (Table 7.9). Both manufacturers of implanted pumps used for pain have useful patient education booklets. Patients and their support persons must also view and handle the pump; we have had a few patients refuse treatment when they felt the weight of the pumps.

Patients should be given sufficient opportunity to ask questions. Misconceptions exist regarding the risks and benefits of intrathecal opioids delivered by implanted pumps, and patients may not voice these concerns unless encouraged. A list of commonly asked questions regarding the implanted pump appears in Chapter 3.

■ CASE STUDY

The following case study illustrates the care of patients receiving intrathecal morphine for chronic pain.

Table 7.8. Scales frequently used to measure pain intensity.

Numerical Rating Scale

(No pain) 0 1 2 3 4 5 6 7 8 9 10 (Worst pain imaginable)

Adjectival rating scale
  No pain
  Mild pain
  Uncomfortable
  Distressing
  Horrible
  Excruciating

Visual analog scale |————————————————| (Worst pain
  (No pain)   imaginable)

Pain History

L.B. presented to the neurosurgery service at age 67 with a longstanding history of postpolio syndrome and severe osteoporosis. She experienced severe, intermittent low back pain, described as "throbbing" in quality, that had existed for several years but was now worsening. No radiculopathy was noted. The patient also experienced generalized joint pain, particularly in the hands and knees, consistent with arthritis, but was not distressed as a result of this pain. The patient was confined to a wheelchair and had a home aide for assistance with basic hygiene, meal preparation, and care of the apartment. L.B. was clearly an intelligent, well-read individual, who attended many lecture series at local museums and universities prior to the worsening of her pain. She was very frustrated that the pain prevented her from these types of leisure activities. Additionally, despite the physical disability, L.B. expressed interest in part-time employment or volunteer work, and anger that she could not participate owing to the severe pain.

Medication History

L.B. had been given nonsteroidal antiinflammatory drugs for pain, but had experienced gastrointestinal pain with the sequential use of several of these drugs. Weak opioids, such as codeine and hydrocodone, produced sedation and severe constipation, and were ineffective in relieving the pain. Stronger opioids, such as oral morphine, led to dysphoria, significant sedation unrelieved by increased caffeine intake, and constipation unaffected by large doses of laxatives and stool softeners. Several tricyclic antidepressants caused urinary retention and did not relieve the

Table 7.9. Patient teaching instructions: implanted pumps for pain.

Before pump implantation

You will be interviewed by your doctor or nurse regarding the events that led to the pain. After the interview, you will be examined for any possible physical changes. It is very helpful to bring in any records from previous hospitalizations and other physicians you have seen. Also bring to the meeting any X-rays, CT scans, or MRIs, including the actual film and diagnostic radiologist's report. Finally, bring pill bottles from the medicines you take now and a list of any past medicines you have taken for pain.

After meeting with your doctor or nurse, you will be asked to make an appointment with the psychologist who works with people in pain. Pain affects all parts of your life, including psychological function. The psychologist will interview you and give you some tests to complete at a later time. The purpose of this visit is to help ascertain whether you need assistance in this area and potential nondrug therapies that might help in relieving your pain.

Screening

At a later point, you may be admitted to the hospital and may be given a brief trial of morphine into the area around your spinal canal (epidural or intrathecal space). This might be a one-time injection into the spinal area, or a temporary catheter may be placed to deliver continuous medication. If you obtain good pain relief without significant side effects, the pump may then be implanted.

Pump implantation

You should have nothing to eat or drink starting at midnight before surgery. An IV will be placed to give you some fluids and antibiotics. During surgery you will be awake, but sleepy. The doctors will give you as much medicine as needed to keep you from experiencing pain. Be sure to let them know if you feel any discomfort.

You will have two incisions, one over the abdomen for the pump and one small incision over your lower back where the catheter is inserted. After surgery you will return to your room. Some patients experience a little pain from the incisions. Your doctor will order medicine to treat this, but you must let the nurses know if you are having any pain. Holding a pillow or folded towel over the abdominal incision may be helpful, especially when you cough or walk.

(Continued)

Table 7.9. (*Continued*)

Discharge

   Most patients go home 1 or 2 days after surgery; some need to stay a little longer. Be sure to bring loose-fitting clothes, such as sweatpants, for the trip home. You can take a sponge bath while the sutures are in place, but no baths or showers. The incision can be open to the air, but if this is uncomfortable, you can cover the area with a gauze pad. Use as little tape as possible to prevent skin irritation. Call _____-_____-_____ if you notice redness, swelling, bleeding, drainage from the incisions, or if you develop a high fever (more than 101.5°F).

   Once you are home and return to a more normal routine, keep track of how much pain you have (1–10; 0 means "no pain," 10 means "the worst pain imaginable") and how many medicines you take for pain. Bring this information with you to your next visit.

Follow-up care

   You will need to see your doctor and nurse approximately 1 week to 10 days after surgery. At this time the sutures will be removed. The dose may be adjusted based on how you did at home, and the pump may also be refilled. The frequency of refills depends on how much medicine you receive. Call _____-_____-_____ if you need further adjustments in your dose.

   If you are taking additional oral medicines for pain, never let the number of pills get too low. Always have at least a 5-day supply.

   Call _____ at _____-_____-_____ for appointments, questions, or other concerns.

Emergencies

   For emergencies, such as fever, drainage or bleeding from the pump, difficulty breathing or urinating, or other problems, call _____ at _____-_____-_____ .

Questions

_____

_____

_____

_____

_____

_____

pain. Anticonvulsants, specifically carbamazepine, created liver enzyme changes. Nerve blocks were not indicated because of the bilateral nature of the pain, and steroid injections were ineffective.

Screening

L.B. underwent placement of an epidural catheter with an infusion of 0.3 mg morphine per hour (concentration of morphine is routinely 0.1

mg/mL infused at a rate of 1 to 12 mL/h). She experienced significant pruritus, was given diphenhydramine, and became sedated. For these reasons, she chose not to have the pump implanted at that time and was discharged on oral opioids. Several months later, she returned for increasing complaints of pain and side effects associated with the oral opioids. Although she again developed pruritus, she obtained excellent pain relief during the epidural screening and elected to have the Synchro-Med pump implanted.

Dosing

The initial dose of intrathecal morphine was 0.5 mg/d; however, after several days the dose was reduced to 0.33 mg/d. The infusion stabilized at this dose for approximately 1 year. At that time L.B. experienced gradually increasing pain, and the dose was titrated upward in 10% to 25% increments. At 1, 2, 3, and 4 years after implant the daily doses were 0.3 mg/d, 2.4 mg/d, 3.3 mg/d, and 3.3 mg/d, respectively. The patient has not required emergency room admission for pain, an event that occurred sporadically prior to pump implantation. Additionally, she now volunteers 2 days each week teaching illiterate adults how to read. She states she feels "useful" and overall generally pleased with her health at this time. She has experienced no side effects from the intrathecal morphine.

■ CONCLUSION

The effect of pain on an individual's life can be disastrous. Pharmacologic and nonpharmacologic interventions can be useful in relieving pain in the majority of patients. When patients experience unrelieved pain or significant side effects from analgesics, intraspinal opioids delivered via implanted infusion pumps can serve as an effective alternative.

Careful patient selection and screening are essential. Dose titration begins after surgery and continues throughout therapy. Supplemental analgesics, including opioids, may be necessary. Sudden changes in dose requirements signal system malfunction or the development of new pain problems, either of which requires investigation. Adverse effects associated with intraspinal opioids include those seen immediately after initiating the infusion and problems that occur after longer-term delivery. Ongoing patient education is essential, beginning during initial meetings with the patient and continuing during the course of therapy.

Although new agents are on the horizon, morphine currently is the only approved opioid for delivery via SynchroMed or Infusaid pumps. The need for alternative agents is great, particularly for patients who do not obtain pain relief from opioids or who develop side effects to these drugs.

8

Mechanical System Complications

The mechanical system refers to both the pump and the catheter. System complications related to the drug pump include overinfusion or underinfusion of the drug. However, the vast majority of complications are related to the catheter.[19,118,178] Specifically, the catheter may kink, dislodge, tear, or fibrose.[179] Treatment of a system complication requires surgical intervention in almost every case.

Reasons to assess the system for possible complications may include abrupt change in drug effect, inadequate drug effect despite increasing dose over time, or an inconsistent drug effect. Table 8.1 includes possible system complications and methods to assess them. Methods to assess the problems will be described in more detail.

■ ASSESSMENT OF SYSTEM COMPLICATIONS

Because of the variation in pumps and catheters, only a general assessment of the mechanical system will be presented in this chapter. Technical knowledge of the specific mechanical system is required to deliver the drug safely. Specific calculations and measurements can be found in the manufacturers' manuals since there are several different pump and catheter models. *It must be stressed that assessing the system may entail complex procedures including delivering a bolus and flushing or programming an imaging solution into either the access port or the inlet of the pump reservoir. Because there is a potential for overdose while performing these procedures, the clinician must be aware of the specific concentration and volumes in both the catheter and the pump.*

Identifying a system complication may be obvious when a patient has an abrupt change in spasticity or pain. A more complex situation occurs when the change is subtle or sporadic. The reason for this change may be

Table 8.1. Potential Delivery System Complications and Possible Methods of Assessment.

Possible system complication	Possible methods to assess complication
Catheter	
• Kink/angulation	• More residual volume than expected in drug reservoir • Response to bolus may vary; usually no response • May be noticeable on X-ray or imaging study
• Dislodgment/ disconnection	• No discrepancy in reservoir volume • No response to bolus • Obvious on X-ray
• Hole, tear, or puncture	• No discrepancy in reservoir volume • May be difficult to detect; tends to mimic pattern of tolerance • Verify CSF drug levels from CSF
• Fibrosis	• May have more volume than expected in drug reservoir • Response to bolus may vary • Obvious on imaging study
• Migration out of space	• No response to bolus • X-ray • CT scan • Imaging study
• Difficulty accessing the side port	• Try rotating needle 90° • Reenter with a new needle • Assure CSF back flow (should test + for glucose)
Pump	
• Battery depletion*	• More volume than expected in drug reservoir if battery significantly depleted • "Low battery alarm" should be audible and seen on pump status screen of the programmer
• Underinfusion or stall	• More residual volume than expected in reservoir • May X-ray motor to verify*

(Continued)

Table 8.1. (*Continued*)

Possible system complication	Possible methods to assess complication
Pump	
• Overinfusion	• Clinical signs of overdose may occur • Less residual volume than expected in reservoir
• Inability to access reservoir	• Pump may have been inverted at implantation or spontaneously • Reposition the pump by manual or surgical manipulation • Also may be due to seroma, infections, or obesity (in extreme cases of obesity access may require fluoroscopy)

*Designated for programmable pump.

more difficult to discern and may not necessarily signify a system problem. For example, physiological and psychosocial factors (refer to Chapters 6 and 7) may also cause an inadequate drug effect and should be thoroughly assessed. Tolerance may also be one reason for an insufficient drug effect (refer to Chapters 6 and 7) and should be suspected if the physiological, psychosocial, and mechanical system assessment is negative. Human error may occur during the surgical, programming, or refilling procedure, which may account for a change in drug effect and may lead to serious adverse effects.

Complications in either the catheter or the pump may cause a change in delivery of medication to the intrathecal space which results in clinical symptoms. These symptoms can be abrupt, intermittent, or gradual and can range from mild to severe. An excess delivery of medication may cause adverse effects, possibly overdose, whereas an ineffective amount may result in increased pain or spasticity and potentially withdrawal symptoms.

Some methods to assess system complications can be done quite simply, such as comparing actual reservoir volumes with the expected reservoir volumes and observing a drug effect from a bolus. More extensive methods include imaging studies for visual assessment of catheter placement, drug flow, or rotor movement. Finally, an elaborate method to assess levels of medication in the CSF may be done, but this is rarely needed. The easiest, least invasive, and least expensive techniques are performed first.

A typical sequence of assessment includes assessment of the reservoir volume, assessment of the patient's response to a bolus, visual assessment of the system and, in rare cases, detection of medication levels in the CSF. These methods to assess system complications will be discussed.

Assessment of Reservoir Volume

Each drug pump model has a specific reservoir volume that needs to be identified for several reasons. Overpressurization may destroy a programmable drug pump; an empty or near empty reservoir volume may cause a decrease in drug effect; and a discrepancy in volume may indicate a complication. Although rare, overpressurization of a programmable pump may lead to overdose, in which case an empty reservoir may lead to withdrawal of medications, and a discrepancy may be an indicator of a system complication.

Overpressurization of Reservoir in Programmable Drug Pump

The reservoir holds an exact volume which is indicated in the manual. Knowledge of this volume is of great importance since overfill can cause damage to the pump by overpressurizing the tubing in the pump, possibly leading to a significant or fatal overdose. To prevent such an occurrence, a pressure monitor device, included in the refill kit, should be used. Also, before the medication is instilled into the pump, any remaining drug should be withdrawn and accounted for.

Low Reservoir Volume

A low reservoir volume, though not considered a complication, may cause a decrease in drug effect in both the SynchroMed and Infusaid pumps. In the SynchroMed pumps, the accuracy of drug delivery decreases by approximately 15% when the reservoir volume is down to 2 mL. In a recent case report,[140] a patient developed an acute withdrawal syndrome when the pump reservoir was empty. The alarm volume was set at 0.5mL; upon arrival to the hospital the telemetry reading was 0.3 ml and the actual volume that was aspirated from the reservoir was 0. Accurate measurement of drug volume is significant; however, there is always a margin of error. We typically use 2 mL as the alarm volume to preclude diminished drug effect due to low reservoir volume. If this diminished effect is noticeable to the patient even with 2 mL remaining in the reservoir, the alarm volume is then programmed to 3 or 4 mL.

In the Infusaid pump, the flow is approximately 4% slower at lower volumes. When the pump is allowed to operate with a volume of 4 mL or less, the variation in flow will be even greater. It is not recommended that a pump be allowed to operate below this minimum reservoir volume. A change in flow rate may be due to geographical altitude, drug-related variables (such as concentration and viscosity), or temperature. The manufacturer has developed a Performance Data Sheet specific to each pump to determine the actual percentage of change in flow rate occurring with changes in altitude (Fig. 8.1).

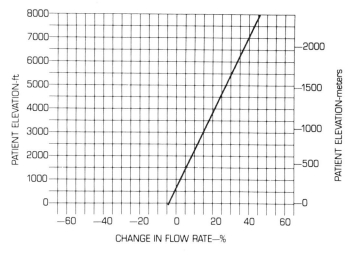

Figure 8.1. Example of the specific Performance Data Sheet which accompanies each pump for the actual percentage of change in flow rate due to increased geographic attitude. If a patient moves to a different altitude, a change in flow rate may occur. Also, pump flow rates may increase significantly during airline flight and cause intolerable adverse effects that may be best managed by refilling the pump with preservative-free 0.9% normal saline for the duration of the flight. (Courtesy of Pfizer Infusaid, Inc, Norwood, Mass.)

Volume Discrepancy in Reservoir

The actual volume in the reservoir, measured by aspirating the fluid from the pump, is compared with the expected volume (calculated by the computer in the programmable pumps and by hand in the nonprogrammable pumps). Both volumes should be documented when the reservoir is accessed. A discrepancy, or major difference, between the two volumes may signify a refill error or a system complication. A change in a patient's clinical effect may confirm either complication.

Overinfusion of the pump may have occurred if the actual volume measured is *less* then the expected volume, especially if the patient is experiencing symptoms of drug overdose. If the actual volume is *greater* than the expected volume, a system complication may be occurring, including pump stall (rare), battery depletion, catheter fibrosis, or, more commonly, a catheter kink. Patients' symptoms may include increased pain or spasticity. See Table 8.2 for guidelines to calculate the percentage of error in the programmable pumps. Errors of <75% would signify an underinfusion, whereas errors of >125% would signify overinfusion.

Table 8.2. Calculating the percentage of error in the SynchroMed pump (Medtronic, Inc., Minneapolis, Minn).

$$\% \text{ Error} = \frac{\text{Expected residual volume (mL)} - \text{actual residual volume (mL)}}{\text{Expected volume (mL)}} \times 100$$

$$\% \text{ Error} = \frac{\text{Expected residual volume} - \text{actual residual volume}}{\text{Previous refill volume} - \text{expected residual volume}} \times 100$$

Example:

$$\% \text{ Error} = \frac{2 \text{ mL} - 9 \text{ mL}}{18 \text{ mL} - 2 \text{ mL}} \times 100 = 44\% \text{ underinfusion}$$

(Reprinted with permission from Medtronic[16])

For nonprogrammable pumps, a change in flow rate of 8% would signify a system complication. Another way to determine if the drug is being delivered accurately is to assess the patient's response to a bolus.

Assessment of Patient Response to a Bolus

One way to verify if the medication is reaching the intrathecal space, or if the patient is receiving an appropriate effect from the drug, is to deliver a single bolus. The bolus can give a specific amount of medication either by programming a set dose or by injecting drug into the side port. This dose should be effective enough to achieve a response to the drug, but not enough to cause an overdose. To avoid overdose, it is essential to review the patient's previous response to the screening dose(s).

After the bolus is given, the patient needs to be assessed within 1 to 2 hours for efficacy and possible side effects. No response to the bolus may indicate a mechanical problem such as catheter kink, dislodgment, disconnection, fibrosis, or pump stall. Further work-up may be needed to diagnoses a more specific problem.

A positive response to the bolus does not necessarily mean there are no mechanical problems. There is a possibility, with a hole or partial kink, that the medication may still reach the tip of the catheter, giving the patient a good or fair response. Radiographic or imaging studies may be needed if the patient does not have an adequate response to the bolus however, problems not related to the system should also be considered.

Assessing the reservoir volume and the patient's response to a bolus dose provides valuable information, but does not ascertain where the specific problem is located. Radiographic or imaging studies may be needed to provide this information.

Radiographic and Imaging Studies

Assessment of the system may be needed when a complication is suspected. The methods to assess complications include X-rays, contrast, and radionuclide studies. In a rare instance where the motor of the programmable pump is believed to have failed, X-rays can be used to determine proper rotor rotation. Also, the catheters used with both the programmable and the nonprogrammable pumps are radiopaque, and X-rays can provide excellent images of catheter placement. Contrast and radionuclide studies can also reveal catheter placement and provide valuable information regarding flow of the drug as well.

X-rays

There are two different ways that X-rays can be utilized to diagnose complications in pumps. First, an X-ray of *both* anterior-posterior (AP) and lateral views of the abdominal/thoracic region may be useful in verifying catheter placement. AP and lateral views may show such complications as migration (this may also be seen by CT scan using horizontal cuts but is far more expensive), dislodgment, disconnection, and, more commonly, a kink in the catheter. A kink may not always be easily detected from AP views alone, however, and comparison of AP and lateral views is usually necessary, especially if the kink is in the distal portion of the catheter within the lumbar fascia (which in our experience is more common). In Figure 8.2, X-rays of normal catheter placement, catheter dislodgment, and catheter kink can be seen.

It is essential to explain to the radiology technologist exactly what is needed and the purpose of the test when ordering an X-ray. The following is an example of such an order:

> AP and lateral views of the abdominal/lower thoracic region to verify placement of a radiopaque catheter. Pay close attention to the catheter connected to the pump located in the left lower quadrant, passing around the left side and continuing upward where the tip of the catheter is placed in the lumbar region.

Secondly, X-rays may be used to confirm movement of the rotor of the programmable pump to diagnose underinfusion. This is typically done after a catheter kink has been ruled out. Two X-rays are needed—the first to verify the position of the rotor, and the second to verify the position after a specific amount of medication is bolused via telemetry to move the rotor 90°, or the bolus can be programmed with the rotor movement verified with fluoroscopy (refer to Clinical Reference Guide by Medtronic[16]). Caution should be exercised to avoid an overdose. The X-rays are taken in an AP view and need to be overexposed slightly to get

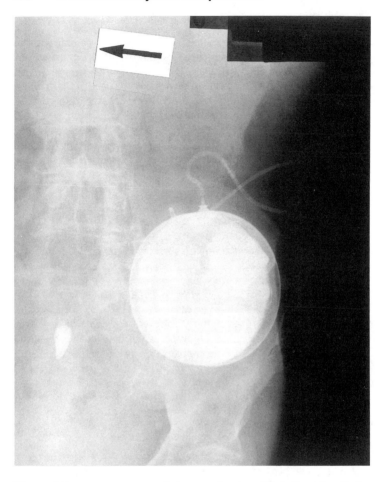

Figure 8.2. (a) Radiograph of a correctly placed intrathecal catheter. Tip resting at approximately the L_1 level.

a good view of the rotor. The views before and after a bolus are compared to see if the rotor has turned 90° (Fig. 8.3).

Although not a complication, a low battery may cause the pump to slow down. Typically, the battery life is 3 to 5 years and the longevity is dose related. A low battery occurrence is noted by an alarm, and/or a low battery message via telemetry appears on the right lower corner of the screen. However, this message may not appear with the onset of diminished battery supply. Low battery life should also be considered as a possibility for underinfusion.

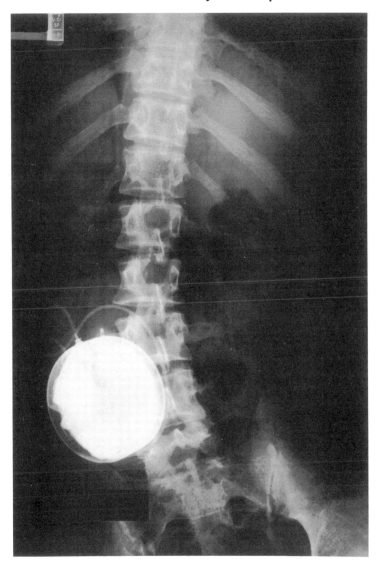

Figure 8.2. (b) Radiograph illustrating the spinal catheter dislodged out of the intrathecal space.

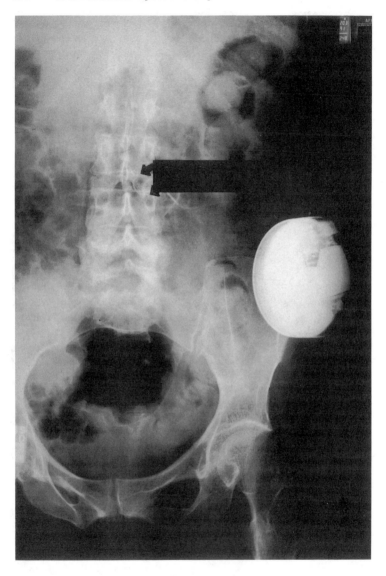

Figure 8.2. (c) Two catheter kinks are present. After this intrathecal catheter was surgically replaced, two holes were noted in the catheter where the kinks occurred.

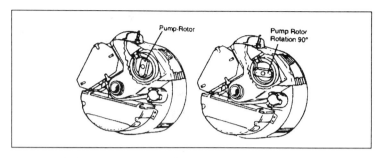

Figure 8.3. This rotor should turn 90° over 45 seconds when an appropriate bolus is calculated and programmed. (Refer to the Clinical Reference Guide by Medtronic[16]) (Courtesy of Medtronic, Minneapolis, Minn.)

Contrast Studies

Radiopaque solution or contrast medium can be used to enhance visualization of the flow of fluid through a catheter. Note that using contrast material that is not indicated for intrathecal administration may result in severe adverse effects.[16]Possible system complications to be identified are catheter kink, dislodgment, fibrosis, or migration out of intrathecal space. Drug pumps with side ports allow direct access to the tip of the catheter, and more importantly, the intrathecal (subarachnoid) space. Because of the potential to overdose the patient when delivering an intrathecal bolus, guidelines are given by the manufacturer regarding specific bolusing procedures.

Approximately 0.5 to 1 mL of medication is aspirated from the side port prior to injection to ensure removal of drug from catheter side port and catheter. Determining the patency of the catheter entails injecting a radiopaque solution such as iopamidol (Isoview), into the side port and viewing the flow under fluoroscopy. If fluoroscopy cannot be used, plain radiograph views of the pump and catheter may also be used.[22] Additionally, contrast media may be used during surgery to view catheter patency (Fig. 8.4). Although this technique is useful, some problems such as a hole within the catheter, may yet be difficult to detect.

Radionuclide Studies

An alternative diagnostic test incorporates the use of a radionuclide study using indium-111 diethylenetriamine pentaacetic acid (DTPA).[180] Although the same system complications can be identified using contrast medium, this technique is especially useful for drug pumps without a side port, since there is no direct access to the CSF.

The indium-111 DTPA is sterile and needs to be ordered a day or 2 ahead of time because of decay. Approximately 250 to 500 μCi in a

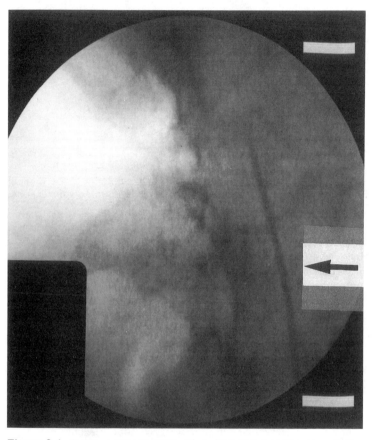

Figure 8.4. C-arm assisted view of a fibrosed intrathecal catheter. Contrast media injected during surgery (Isoview) confirmed the fibrosis since the dye could not flow cephalad.

volume of approximately 0.2 mL is needed. This small amount is injected directly into the central reservoir using sterile technique. In order not to dilute the indium-111 DTPA, the reservoir volume is typically kept around 6 mL.

To obtain useful images, the approximate time needed for the indium to reach the catheter tip and the cisternal CSF must be considered. To determine how many hours are necessary for the indium-111 DTPA to reach the tip of the catheter, the volume in both the pump and the catheter must be calculated. To obtain the flow rate, the concentration of the drug is divided by the hourly dose; this is multiplied by the volume (mL) in both the pump and catheter tubing space to obtain the number of hours necessary for the indium-111 DTPA to reach the catheter tip (Table 8.3).

Table 8.3. Number of Hours it Takes for Indium-111 DTPA to Pass Through the Reservoir Up to Catheter Tip.

$$\frac{\text{Concentration}}{\text{Hourly dose}} \times \text{volume (mL) in pump and catheter tubing space}$$

Equation applicable for both Medtronic programmable pumps and Infusaid constant-flow pumps.

After this is determined, an additional 12 to 24 hours should be added allowing the indium to ascend rostrally to the brain. The exact time may depend on the availability of the patient and scanner; however, after 4 to 5 days the indium may not be detected due to breakdown. The images of the lower, middle, and upper region in posterior projection are obtained with some views overlapping an entire view. Figure 8.5 illustrates normal flow; in contrast, Figure 8.6 illustrates a fibrosed catheter.

Detecting Appropriate Levels of Medication Via CSF Assays

In extreme cases, a patient may continue to have an ineffective clinical response from the medication and have no detected system complication. If the decrease in clinical effect is not abrupt, or if tolerance to the medication is suspected, evaluation of appropriate medication levels in the CSF may be warranted.

Through analysis of lumbar CSF levels by high-performance liquid chromatography (HPLC), the amount of medication within the CSF can be verified (refer to Table 8.4 for calculating this value).[25] A low value would indicate improper drug levels, suggesting a system complication such as a hole, or improperly diluting or labeling by pharmacy. High or normal levels may suggest that the patient is tolerant to the medication.

■ CONCLUSION

The frequency and types of complications vary; however, most complications are related to the catheter. In the United States monitored clinical trials conducted from 1984 to 1992, 473 patients received intrathecal baclofen through SynchroMed programmable drug pumps. The complication rate related to the system was 19.9% (Table 8.5). In a retrospective survey of 429 patients receiving intrathecal drugs for pain through programmable drug pumps, the system complication rate was 18.8%.[171]

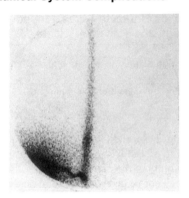

(a) From drug pump up to
         lumbar area.

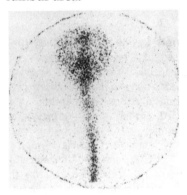

(b) Rostral flow to cistern.

Figure 8.5. (a) Normal flow is observed in this catheter after 48 hours, when indium-111 flow exceeded the tip of the catheter. The bright, round area is the drug pump, and the small bright line to the left of the pump is the catheter tunneled around the side of the body. The vertical line extending from the pump represents the flow of the radioactive dye present in the lumbar and thoracic regions. (b) A second image illustrating indium-111 DTPA ascending to the cisternal level. This is considered a normal indium flow study.

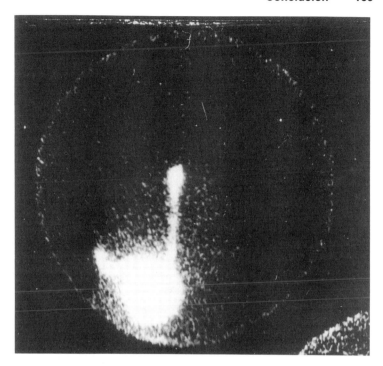

Figure 8.6. An abnormal indium flow study representing a fibrosed catheter. Indium is only visible at the lumbar level, 48 hours after the indium reached the catheter tip.

Table 8.4. Calculation of Expected Drug Concentration in the CSF After Continuous Intrathecal Administration.

Divide the hourly intrathecal drug dose in mg by 30 (the approximate hourly rate of CSF clearance in humans) to determine the approximate amount of drug that should be present in the CSF. Fluid can be obtained through a lumbar tap. This formula is accurate for hydrophilic drugs such as morphine, hydromorphine, and baclofen delivered intrathecally. This formula would not be appropriate for calculating the concentration of drugs such as fentanyl and sufentanyl.

Example: $\dfrac{X \text{ mg/h}}{30} = X$ mg/mL

(Reprinted with permission from Paice and Williams.[40])

Table 8.5. System-related complications* (US clinical studies)

	Number	Percent
Total patients implanted	473	100.0
Patients with system complications[†]	94	19.9
Follow-up (months)		
Mean	21	
Range	0.0–101.5	
SD	19	
Sum	9943.4	
Total Complications	**141**	**97.9[‡]**
Catheter		
Catheter disconnect	3	2.1
Catheter dislodged/migration	14	9.9
Catheter fibrosis	5	3.5
Catheter fracture	24	17.0
Catheter kink/occlusion	52	36.9
Catheter port fracture	1	0.7
Catheter punctured	5	3.5
Connector assembly occlusion/punctured	5	3.5
CSF leak	1	0.7
Lack of effect	3	2.1
Pseudominingocale	2	1.4
Pump		
Alarm malfunction	4	2.8
Pump flipped	1	0.7
Pump motor stall	6	4.3
Pump over/under infusion	3	2.1
Pump overinfusion	5	3.5
Pump telemetry failure	1	0.7
Pump under/no infusion	6	4.3

*Directly attributable to device or occurring more than 60 days postoperatively.
[†]Some patients experienced more than one system complication.
[‡]Percentage is based on total system complications.
(Reprinted with permission from Medtronic, Inc.)

Mechanical system complications may not always be obvious; they may occur overtime and may be quite frustrating when a definite problem cannot be determined (Fig. 8.7). Although not very common, such a situation may necessitate surgical exploration of the mechanical system.[178]

There are several diagnostic procedures that can be performed to assess a system complication. Clinicians need to be proficient when using these procedures, especially since some procedures may cause an overdose if done incorrectly. If surgical intervention is needed, in our experience almost every patient has elected to do so, since many have had a significant positive effect from the drug prior to developing the complication.

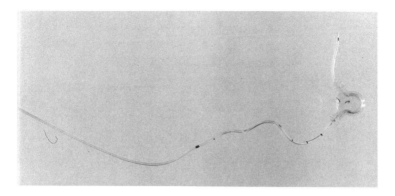

(a)

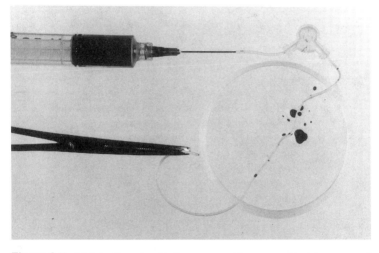

(b)

Figure 8.7. (a) Intrathecal catheter removed from a patient because of two kinks and two holes. When dye is manually injected through the catheter, the holes cannot be detected. (b) The two holes are visualized in the same catheter, but only after one end of the catheter is clamped while the dye is manually injected under pressure. It must be emphasized that tiny holes in intraspinal catheters are extremely difficult to detect with dye studies. Medication may not always escape through the holes unless the hole gets larger from constant kinking. Clinically, the patient may experience intermittent episodes of spasticity.

9

Starting Up a Program

Prior to beginning a program using implanted drug pumps for the delivery of intrathecal drugs, significant coordination must take place. The setting where patients will be followed must be chosen, supplies must be purchased, the appropriate personnel must be convened, policies and tools for documentation must be developed, coordination between other departments must be initiated, and reimbursement strategies must be considered. This chapter will alert clinicians to these considerations along with providing useful tools to assist with these efforts.

■ CHOOSE A SETTING FOR FOLLOW-UP CARE

Surgical implantation of drug pumps typically occurs within hospital settings, although financial pressures may increase the number of surgeries conducted in outpatient centers. Long-term follow-up, including assessment, refills, and dose titration may take place in physicians' offices, outpatient clinics, or even in the home. If caring for patients in outpatient offices or clinics, rooms should be designed for the special needs of these patients. Large rooms and wide doorways are necessary to accommodate the needs of patients in motorized wheelchairs. Examination tables should be easily accessible for immobilized patients with neurologic disorders or pain. Equipment for monitoring vital signs is also needed.

In addition to an appropriate setting, other essential components, such as 24-hour coverage, must be planned. Answering services must be available, and patients must know what numbers to contact, so that in case of emergencies the appropriate staff can be contacted. Emergency equipment should be accessible. If not connected with a hospital or if emergency equipment is not easily available, these supplies should be purchased: an airway, and Ambu bag, intravenous catheters and fluids, and several vials of naloxone. Some centers not in close proximity to a hospital may wish also to have cardiac monitors and physostigmine available in case of baclofen overdose.

■ OBTAIN SUPPLIES

The necessary supplies must be obtained prior to the implantation of the first pump. This ensures continuous and safe care. For example, refill kits must be available for screening and before pumps are implanted in case the device must be accessed immediately after surgery. Extra syringes, needles, sterile gloves, and other supplies should be available (Table 9.1) If using programmable pumps, the programmer must be obtained. Keep in mind that because a programmer is needed during the surgical implantation, a second programmer will be necessary if outpatients are to be refilled during this time, or such patients should be scheduled when surgeries are not planned. Because the cost of the programmers is not minor, the purchaser needs to be determined before the first pump is implanted. In some centers, the implanting physician purchases the programmer, particularly if his/her practice will be reimbursed for refills. In other settings, the hospital or outpatient center may pay for, and own, the programmer.

Table 9.1. Recommended Supplies
for Refilling Implanted Pumps.

Refill kits
22-gauge noncoring needles
Povidone-iodine swabs
Alcohol wipes
0.2-μm filters
Adhesive dressings
Syringes
Three-way stopcocks
Preservative-free saline
Sterile gloves
Suture/staple removal kits

■ CONVENE PERSONNEL

An interdisciplinary approach is necessary when caring for patients receiving this technology (Fig. 9.1). Because these health care professionals may devote only part of their time to the care of these patients, they must be fully educated in the use of this therapy. Psychologists; physical, vocational, and occupational therapists; social workers; and many others have much to contribute to the care of patients with implanted pumps, but to do so requires that they understand the rationale for the therapy. We recommend a regular meeting of all staff to communicate concerns and develop a plan of care.

To foster knowledge regarding the treatment of pain and neurological disorders, team members are advised to join professional organizations that provide current information at seminars and conferences and through scientific journals. Resources for those working in the areas of spasticity and pain are included in Appendices 3.2, 4.2, and 5.

In addition to health care professionals, secretarial services are essential for scheduling patient appointments as well as managing correspondence with other clinicians and third-party payers. The secretarial support persons can assist with triaging phone calls and messages,

Interdisciplinary Care

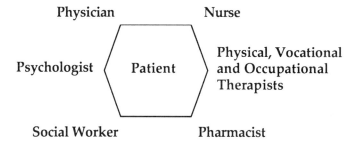

Figure 9.1. Interdisciplinary approach to painh management. Many health care professionals, including nurses, physicians, pharmacists, psychologists, therapists, pastoral care personnel, rehabilitation specialists, and others, can assist in the care of persons with chronic intractable pain. Each brings his/her own contribution; however, communication is essential.

developing a system of charting, purchasing necessary supplies, and other activities.

■ DEVELOP POLICIES AND PROCEDURES

A policy and procedure should be available to guide the nursing care of these patients while in the hospital (see Appendix 2). Other departments, such as the pharmacy and emergency room, may wish to develop policies for the preparation of the medications and urgent care of the patient. Because these policies must often be approved by various committees, it is essential that they be developed before the first patient is admitted for implantation.

■ GENERATE TOOLS FOR DOCUMENTATION

Documentation is essential, not only for ensuring continuity of care, but also for legal concerns. Forms should include vital information regarding the refill, the delivery system's performance, the drug dosage, and the patient's response to therapy. Samples of such forms are included in Figures 9.2 through 9.5. Documenting the prescription of supplemental medication helps track the use of these medications over time (Fig. 9.6). Brief comments or ancedotal notes are helpful for documenting potential problems with the delivery system or dose adjustments.

■ COORDINATE ACTIVITIES OF OTHER DEPARTMENTS

Operating Room Staff

Those working in the operating room must understand the specific recommendations for pump preparation provided by each manufacturer. Videotapes, manuals, and posters are available for their use. The clinicians caring for these patients after surgery may wish to provide inservices to OR staff as a mechanism not only to improve knowledge, but also to foster communication and the team approach.

Staff responsible for ordering supplies in the OR must be provided with the names and telephone numbers of the pump manufacturers. They should be instructed regarding how many pumps and catheters must be ordered, including specific model numbers. When using continuous flow

Patient Hospital No. _____   Patient Initials _____ _____ _____   Pump Serial Number _ _ _ _ _ _ _ _

Date Pump Implant _____ / _____ / _____
Month   Day   Year

FOLLOW-UP DATA   Form 4

A. Pump Refilled   ☐ Yes   ☐ No   Evaluation Date _____ / _____ / _____
Month   Day   Year

Actual Residual Volume (ml) _____   Refill Drug _____
Programmer Residual Volume (ml) _____   Lot Number _____
Refill Volume_____

B. Change in program   ☐ Yes   ☐ No

Drug Concentration: _____ ☐ µg per ml   Dose: _____ ☐ µg   ☐ per day
☐ mg per ml   ☐ mg   ☐ per hour

Mode: ☐ Continuous   ☐ Complex   ☐ Bolus Delay   ☐ Bolus   ☐ Off

C. Procedures performed at this follow-up: ☐ µg

☐ Access Port Flush   ☐ Pump Bolus dose: _____ ☐ mg   ☐ Other, specify: _____

D. Neurological Assessment

Rigidity (1-5)	L	R	Voluntary Muscle Movement	L	R
Hip Abduction			Upper Extremities	☐ None	☐ None
Hip Flexion				☐ Limited	☐ Limited
Knee Flexion				☐ Normal	☐ Normal
Ankle Dorsiflexion			Lower Extremities	☐ None	☐ None
Spasms (0-4)				☐ Limited	☐ Limited
				☐ Normal	☐ Normal

E. Functional Assessment

Primary Mode of Mobility:
☐ wheelchair   ☐ ambulatory   ☐ ambulatory with walker   ☐ bedridden   ☐ other _____

Urinary Management		**Bowel Management**	
☐ Normal	☐ Intermittent Catheter	☐ Suppository	☐ Normal
☐ Indwelling Catheter	☐ Suprapubic	☐ Digital Stimulation	☐ Other: _____
☐ External Catheter	☐ Other: _____		
☐ Reflex without Catheter			

F. Any Concomitant Medication   ☐ Yes   ☐ No

Drug	Daily Dose	Indications	

G. Adverse Effect or System Complication   ☐ Yes   ☐ No   If yes, complete Forms 5 and/or 6

H. Comments: _____
_____
_____

INVESTIGATOR SIGNATURE _____

Figure 9.2. Form to document the use of Lioresal Intrathecal by the Medtronic pump. (*Reprinted with permission from Medtronic, Minneapolis, Minn.*)

pumps, the approximate flow rate desired should also be specified. These staff people may be advised that as soon as a product is used, a replacement is ordered. Additionally, because catheters have the potential to be damaged or to malfunction, we recommend having at least two or three extra catheters available at all times. When using programmable pumps, however, it is best not to have too many in stock if few patients are scheduled for implant, since the battery may be depleted over time. Furthermore, some surgeons may wish to use other equipment, and the OR staff and purchasing personnel must be aware of these needs.

BACLOFEN FLOW SHEET Patient Initials___ __ __

Implant Date_____ Pump Serial #__ __ __ __ __ __ - - - - -

Meds_____

Date (mo/day/yr)	/ /		/ /		/ /		/ /	
Refilled?	☐ Yes	☐ No	☐ Yes	☐ No	☐ Yes	☐ No	☐ Yes	☐ No
Refill Volume	___ _ . ___ ml		___ _ . ___ ml		___ : ___ ml		___ _ . ___ ml	
Actual Residual Volume	___ _ . ___ ml		___ _ . ___ ml		___ _ . ___ ml		___ _ . ___ ml	
Programmer Residual Volume	___ _ . ___ ml		___ _ . ___ ml		___ _ . ___ ml		___ _ . ___ ml	
Drug/lot #:								
Concentration in Pump (µg/ml)	/ml		/ml		/ml		/ml	
Dose (µg/hour)								
Total Daily Dose (µg)								
Mode of Infusion	☐ Continuous ☐ Cont./Complex ☐ Bolus		☐ Continuous ☐ Cont./Complex ☐ Bolus		☐ Continuous ☐ Cont./Complex ☐ Bolus		☐ Continuous ☐ Cont./Complex ☐ Bolus	
Rigidity (1-5 Ashworth Scale)	L	R	L	R	L	R	L	R
Hip Abduction								
Hip Flexion								
Knee Flexion								
Ankle Dorsiflexion								
Spasms (0-4)								
Reflex								
Notes								
System Complications	☐ Yes(See Form5) ☐ No		☐ Yes(See Form 5) ☐ No		☐ Yes(See Form 5) ☐ No		☐ Yes(See Form 5) ☐ No	
Adverse Effects	☐ Yes(See Form 6) ☐ No		☐ Yes(See Form 6) ☐ No		☐ Yes(See Form 6) ☐ No		☐ Yes(See Form 6) ☐ No	

Investigator Signature_____

Figure 9.3. Another Lioresal Intrathecal documentation form.

Pharmacy Personnel

The pharmacy staff in the OR, inpatient setting, and outpatient center must be prepared for the need for new medications. If the pharmacists involved choose to use commercially available preparations, then these supplies must be ordered and available prior to the first implantation. Because emergencies may occur, additional supplies should always be accessible. If medications are to be reconstituted from tablets, policies must be developed and approved. We strongly encourage the use of laminar flow hoods and 0.2-μm filters when drawing up solutions from vials or during reconstitution of drug.

Particularly within the outpatient setting, a mechanism must be in place for how the medication will be obtained. Our refills occur in an outpatient center that contains an outpatient pharmacy. We call in the prescription several hours prior to the patient's appointment to allow the pharmacist time to prepare the medication. The patient stops at the pharmacy prior to coming to the office, picks up the medication, and brings it to our office several floors above the pharmacy.

In 10 states, the use of multiple copy prescriptions is mandatory to obtain schedule II drugs, including morphine. Physicians who live in these states who will be responsible for the delivery of intraspinal opioids by implanted pump must obtain these prescription pads from their state prior to beginning this program of therapy.

Nursing Staff

If patients are to be admitted to the inpatient setting during screening or for postoperative care, we recommend that one unit be designated for their care. This allows the nursing staff to develop a level of expertise in caring for these patients that occurs after repeated exposure to this therapy. Inservices can be provided along with written teaching tools. If patients are to be discharged to long-term care facilities, the staff at these centers need to have beginning knowledge regarding the pump and its function, skin care, and potential adverse drug effects. They must also have emergency telephone numbers available so that if problems occur, the appropriate personnel are contacted.

■ REIMBURSEMENT STRATEGIES

Developing a plan for billing prior to the first implantation is essential. Both manufacturers of implanted pumps provide written information regarding the codes that can be used to bill for services and offer reimbursement specialists who can offer assistance with billing (Table 9.2). New CPT codes to be used for billing for refills are under consideration; check the most up-to-date manual of codes or contact the reimbursement specialists for assistance.

Many third-party payers require additional information when considering reimbursement issues. Preapproval is absolutely essential, and letters of medical necessity may be required. Therefore, secretarial and billing support services are essential to the successful function of this program.

FORM 2a
FOLLOW-UP - Single Agent
Medtronic SynchroMed Infusion System

Patient Name _____

Implant Date _____   Date of Follow-up _____
              mo   day   yr

Follow-up Physician _____   Pump Serial No. _ _ _ _ _ _ _ _ _ _

A. **Pump Refilled** ☐ Yes   ☐ No.   If no, please go on to Section B.

    Actual Residual Vol. ___ ___•___ ml   Refill Drug _____

    Programmer Residual Vol. ___ ___•___ ml   Refill Vol. ___ ___•___ ml

B. **Change in Drug, Concentration or Prescription** ☐ Yes   ☐ No
   If no, go on to Section C.

    Drug Concentration _____   ☐ ug   ☐ per ml
                                    ☐ mg
                                    ☐ units

    Programmed Dose or Rate _____ ☐ ug ☐ mg ☐ units ☐ ul ☐ ml **per hour**

                             _____ ☐ ug ☐ mg ☐ units ☐ ul ☐ ml **per day**

    Mode: ☐ Continuous   ☐ Complex   ☐ Bolus Delay   ☐ Bolus   ☐ Off

C. **Programmer Model No.**   ☐ 8800   ☐ 8810   ☐ 8820   ☐ Other: _____

D. **Complications, System Related:**   ☐ Yes   ☐ No
   If yes, please describe in Comments section.

E. **Complications, Drug Related:**   ☐ Yes   ☐ No
   If yes, please describe treatment plan in Comments section.
                        Nausea & vomiting   ☐
                        Pruritus   ☐
                        Sedation   ☐
                        Urinary retention   ☐
                        Motor weakness   ☐
                        Sensory loss   ☐
                        Constipation   ☐
                        Edema   ☐

Figure 9.4. Flow sheet allows documentation of pain, analgesic use, and pump performance when using SynchroMed pump.

■ CONCLUSION

Planning is absolutely critical to the success of any program, particularly one as complex as caring for patients with implanted drug pumps. The appropriate personnel and equipment must be mobilized, and policies must be in place. Each member's role must be clear to the other team members and, most importantly, to the patient. Communication and planning are essential.

F. **Procedure(s) performed at this follow-up:** ☐ Access Port Flush ☐ Pump Bolus
☐ Other _____

G. **Pain Score (0-10):** Average _____ Right now _____ Least _____ Worst _____

H. Supplemental analgesics
_____
_____
_____

I. Comments: _____
_____
_____
_____
_____
_____
_____
_____
_____
_____
_____
_____
_____
_____
_____
_____
_____
_____
_____
_____

Signature _____

Figure 9.4 (*continued*)

INFUSAID CONSTANT FLOW PUMP

REFILL WORKSHEET

Patient Name _____   Serial Number _____

Date of Implant_____   Model Number _____

Catheter Location _____   Calibrated Flow Rate _____

Pump Pocket Location _____   Reservoir Capacity_____

Date _____ Refill Interval _____   Refill Volume _____

Returned Volume _____   Infusate_____

Infused Volume _____   Infusate Concentration _____

Calculated Flow Rate (ml/day) _____Calculated Daily Dose _____

Comments _____

_____

Signature _____

Date _____ Refill Interval _____   Refill Volume _____

Returned Volume _____   Infusate_____

Infused Volume _____   Infusate Concentration _____

Calculated Flow Rate (ml/day) _____Calculated Daily Dose _____

Comments _____

_____

Signature _____

Date _____ Refill Interval _____   Refill Volume _____

Returned Volume _____   Infusate_____

Infused Volume _____   Infusate Concentration _____

Calculated Flow Rate (ml/day) _____Calculated Daily Dose _____

Comments _____

_____

Signature _____

Figure 9.5. Refill worksheet for documentation when using the Infusaid pump. (*Reprinted with permission by Pfizer Infusaid.*)

INSTRUCTIONS

1. Calibrated Flow Rate
   Found on the Performance Data Sheet which accompanies each pump. This rate is preset at the factory.

2. Refill Interval
   Elapsed time since the last refill procedure (the present date minus the date of the last refill).

3. Returned Volume
   Volume returned into the syringe barrel when the pump is emptied.

   NOTE: The refill kit syringe barrel is precalibrated to account for refill tubing volume (.5 ml).

4. Infused Volume
   Total amount of drug infused over the refill cycle (the reservoir volume from the previous cycle minus the returned volume from this cycle).

5. Calculated Flow Rate (ml/day)
   Daily infusion rate of the pump (the infused volume divided by the refill interval).

6. Refill Volume
   Volume in the syringe of new infusate.

   NOTE: Pump reservoir volumes:
   Models 100, 400: 50 mls

7. Infusate
   Drug, concentration, type of diluent, etc...

   NOTE: If dead space equation is used, the syringe drug concentration will be different from the pump drug concentration. Both should be noted on the worksheet.

8. Calculated Daily Dose
   Daily dose of drug administered by the pump (the drug concentration (mg/ml) multiplied by pump flow rate (ml/day)).

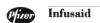

Infusaid

Infusaid, Inc., 1400 Providence Highway, Norwood, MA 02062   Tel 1 800 451 1050   617 769 8330   Fax 617 769 0072 Telex 92 4343

42254
Rev NR   Copyright 1991 by Infusaid Inc

Figure 9.5 (*continued*)

Supplemental Drug Use: Ordering Schedule

Name: _____

Date Ordered	Drug (dose, route, frequency)	#

Figure 9.6. Supplemental drug order form allows the clinician to track the use of oral analgesics.

Table 9.2. Reinbursement Information.

Infusaid, Inc.
Reimbursement Services
Monday to Friday   8 AM to 5:30 PM EST; (800) 451-1050

Medtronic, Inc.
Comprehensive Reimbursement Assistance
Monday to Friday   8 AM to 5 PM CST; (800) 328-0810

10

Current Controversies and Future Applications

■ CONTROVERSIES

Cost

Although administering intraspinal medications such as morphine for pain and baclofen for spasticity have proven to be dramatically successful therapies, controversy still surrounds the high-tech therapy employing a chronic infusion of medications into the spine. Surgically implanting the drug delivery system is invasive, subjecting patients to the typical risks of surgery, but the delivery system is not permanent, allowing alternative methods of treatment to be explored. In addition, motor function is not compromised with this procedure. The cost of the therapy including hospitalization, surgery, physician's fees, drug, and long-term management seems expensive; however, a report prepared by Medtronic, and Charles River Associates compared the cost components of intrathecal baclofen to the cost of associated care with and without intrathecal baclofen and support intrathecal baclofen as being cost-effective.[17,181] A cost analysis conducted by Bedder et al. supports treatment of pain beyond 3months' duration with an implanted delivery system (SynchroMed pump) to be more cost-effective than an external pump and epidural catheter.[182] If the cost of the therapy is deterring patients from treatment, then the treatment's potential efficacy should be considered. Screening procedures are currently being simplified and conducted in out-patient settings, which may decrease the cost of the hospitalization and the total cost of the therapy. Successful treatment requires that patients be compliant with follow-up appointments and provide honest information about the drug's efficacy and the delivery system's performance; however, some selected home care agencies are skilled at providing these services to patients in their homes, especially for those who are bedridden.

Ethics

Many ethical issues remain controversial when treating chronically ill or terminally ill patients with high-tech therapies. Obviously, appropriately selected patients benefit greatly from these therapies. On the other hand, some patients and physicians prefer conservative methods of treatment, which must be respected. The emphasis on patient selection is critical and must consider all of the positive and negative issues involving long-term therapy.

■ FUTURE APPLICATIONS

Looking forward to the 21st century, one can imagine how high-tech equipment will affect health care. Drug pumps may be used for many different applications, and smaller, more sophisticated devices are being developed. In the future, pumps may be designed with patient activated parts, enabling greater flexibility with drug delivery. Medication doses may be initiated or changed by telemetry via telephone. Portable programmers are being designed with additional safety mechanisms that may minimize the risk of error and overdose. Experience with chronic, safe infusion of medications such as baclofen and morphine has proven that the intraspinal route is clinically acceptable and that the pharmacokinetics of drugs can be predicted, as with more traditional routes of administration.

Gaining direct access into the CNS by bypassing the BBB permits local drug administration to many new sites of action. New drug applications are directed toward treating neurodegenerative diseases such as amyotrophic lateral sclerosis (ALS) with large molecular agents, namely neurotrophic substances, which may sustain neural function. Other drug applications are directed at treating disorders in which a neurotransmitter is deficient—e.g., Parkinson's disease. New drugs for moderating pain are constantly being investigated. We live in an exciting era in which advances in this technology, along with expanded drug applications, hold promise for the future in treating a multitude of neurologic disorders. Inspired investigators are encouraged to take this concept and explore safer and more efficient ways of providing chronic drug infusions.

References

1. Blackshear PJ. Implantable drug-delivery systems. *Sci Am.* 1979; 241(6):66–73.
2. Graham A, Holohan T. External and implantable infusion pumps. *Health Tech Rev.* 1993; 7:1–29.
3. Noback C, Demarest R. *The Nervous System Introduction and Review.* 2nd ed. New York, NY: McGraw-Hill, Inc., 1977.
4. Paice J, Magolan J. Intraspinal drug therapy. *Nurs Clin North Am.* 1991; 26(2):477–498.
5. Gilman S, Newman S. *Manter and Gatz's Essentials of Clinical Neuroanatomy and Neurophysiology.* Essentials of Medical Education Series.Philadelphia, Pa: F.A. Davis Company; 1987.
6. Snell R. *Clincal Neuroanatomy for Medical Students.* Boston, Mass: Little, Brown and Company; 1980.
7. Barr M, Kiernan J. *The Human Nervous System: An Anatomical Viewpoint.* 5th ed. Philadelphia, Pa: J.B. Lippincott Co.; 1988.
8. Carpenter M. *Core Text of Neuroanatomy.* 3rd ed. Baltimore, Md: Williams and Wilkins; 1985.
9. Lindsley D, Holmes J. *Basic Human Physiology.* New York, NY: Elsevier; 1984: 113–120.
10. Rexed BA. Cytoarchitectonic atlas of the spinal cord in the cat. *J Comp Neurol.* 1954; 100:297–379.
11. Price GW, Wilkin GP, Turnbull MJ, et al. Are baclofen-sensitive $GABA_B$ receptors present on primary afferent terminals of the spinal cord? *Nature.* 1984; 307(5946):71–74.
12. Kandel E, Schwartz J, Jessell T. *Principles of Neural Science.* 3rd ed. New York, NY: Elsevier Science Publishing Co.; 1991.
13. Waldman S. Implantable drug delivery systems: practical considerations. *J Pain Symptom Manage.* 1990; 5(3):169–174.
14. Muller H, Zierski J, Penn R. *Local-Spinal Therapy of Spasticity.* Berlin, Germany: Springer-Verlag; 1988.

15. Infusaid Pfizer. *Clinicians Manual for the Infusaid Constant Flow Implantable Pump (Model 400).* 1992.

16. Medtronic. *Refill for Intraspinal Applications. SynchroMed Infusion System: Clinical Reference Guide.* 1993.

17. Medtronic. *Lioresal Intrathecal Therapy Reference Guide.* Education Department, 1992.

18. Von Roemeling R, Lanning R, Earnes F. MR imaging of patients with implanted drug infusion pumps. *JMRI.* 1991; 1(1):77–81.

19. Coffey RJ, Cahill D, Steers W, et al. Intrathecal baclofen for intractable spasticity of spinal cord origin: results of a long-term multicenter study. *J Neurosurg.* 1993; 78(2):226–232.

20. Abramowicz M. Antimicrobial prophylaxis in surgery. *Med Lett.* 1992; 34(862):5–8.

21. Classen D, Evans R, Pestotnik S, et al. The timing of prophylactic administration of antibiotics and the risk of surgical wound infection. *N Engl J Med.* 1992; 326(5):281–286.

22. Krames E. Intrathecal infusional therapies for intractable pain: patient management guidelines. *J Pain Symptom Manage.* 1993; 8(1):36–46.

23. Barash P, Cullen B, Stoelting R. *Clinical Anesthesia.* 2nd ed. Philadelphia, Pa: Lippincott; 1992.

24. *Physician's Desk Reference.* 48th ed. Montvale, NJ: Medical Economics Data Production Company; 1994.

25. Kroin JS, Penn RD. Cerebrospinal fluid pharmacokinetics of lumbar intrathecal baclofen. In Lakke JPWF, Delhaas EM, and Rutgers AWF (eds). *Parenteral Drug Therapy in Spasticity and Parkinson's Disease.* Carnforth, UK: Parthenon Publishing; 1991: 73–83.

26. Kroin J, Ali A, York M, et al. The distribution of medication along the spinal canal after chronic intrathecal administration. *Neurosurgery.* 1993; 33(2):226–230.

27. Andersen P, Cohen J, Everts E, et al. Intrathecal narcotics for relief of pain from head and neck cancer. *Arch Otolaryngol Head Neck Surg.* 1991;117:1277–1280.

28. Onofrio B, Yaksh T. Long-term pain relief produced by intrathecal morphine infusion in 53 patients. *J Neurosurg.* 1990; 72(2):200–209.

29. North R. Spinal cord compression complicating subarachnoid infusion of morphine: case report and laboratory experience. *Neurosurgery.* 1991; 29(5):778–784.

30. Paice J. Intrathecal morphine infusion for intractable cancer pain: a new use for implanted pumps. *Oncol Nurs Forum.* 1986; 13(3):41–47.

31. Bennett M, Tai Y, Symonds J. Staphylococcal meningitis following Synchromed intrathecal pump implant: a case report. *Pain.* 1994; 56(2):243–244.

32. Guyton AC (ed). *Basic Neuroscience: Anatomy & Physiology* (2nd ed.), Philadelphia, PA: W.B. Saunders Company; 1991; 125.

33. Kroin JS. Intrathecal drug administration: present use and future trends. *Clin Pharmacokinet.* 1992; 22(5):319–326.

34. DeCastro J, Meynadier J, Zenz M. *Regional Opioid Analgesia.* Boston, Mass: Kluwer; 1991.

35. Payne R, Inturrisi CE. CSF distribution of morphine, methadone and sucrose after intrathecal injection. *Life Sci.* 1985; 37(12):1137–1144.

36. Gourlay G, Cherry D, Plummer J, et al. The influence of drug polarity on the absorption of opioid drugs into CSF and subsequent cephalad migration following lumbar epidural administration: applications to morphine and pethidine. *Pain.* 1987; 31(3):292–305.

37. Gourlay G, Murphy T, Plummer J, et al. Pharmacokinetics of fentanyl in lumbar and cervical CSF following lumbar epidural and intravenous administration. *Pain.* 1989; 38(3):253–259.

38. Sandler A, Stringer D, Panos L, et al. A randomized, double-blind comparison of lumbar epidural and intravenous fentanyl infusions for postthoractomy pain relief. *Anesthesiology.* 1992; 77(4): 626–634.

39. McQuay H, Sullivan A, Smallman K, et al. Intrathecal opioids, potency and lipophilicity. *Pain.* 1989; 36(1):111–115.

40. Paice J, Williams A. Intraspinal drugs for pain. In McGuire, D, Yarbro, C, (eds): *Cancer Pain Management.* 2nd ed. Jones & Bartlett. pp 131–158.

41. Plummer J, Cmielewski P, Reynolds G, et al. Influence of polarity on dose-response relationships of intrathecal opioids in rats. *Pain.* 1990; 40(3):339–347.

42. Craig DB, Habib GG Flacid paralysis following obstetrical epidural anesthesia: possible role of benzyl alcohol. *Anesth Analg.* 1977; 56(2):219–221.

43. DuPen S, Ramsey D, Chin S. Chronic epidural morphine and preservative-induced injury. *Anesthesiology.* 1987; 67(6):987–988.

44. Hersh E, Condouris G, Havelin D. Actions of intrathecal chloroprocaine and sodium bisulfite on rat spinal reflex function utilizing a noninvasive technique. *Anesthesiology.* 1990; 72(6):1077–1082.

45. Wang B, Hillman D, Spielholz N, et al. Subarachnoid toxicity of acetone sodium bisulfite antioxidant in tetracaine HC in rabbits. *Anesth Analg.* 1983; 62:289–290.

46. Wang B, Hillman D, Spielholz N, et al. Subarachnoid blockade by sodium metabisulfite. *Reg Anesth.* 1984; 9:45–47.

47. DuPen S, Peterson D, Bogosian A, et al. A new permanent exteriorized epidural catheter for narcotic self-administration to control cancer pain. *Cancer.* 1987; 59(5):986–993.

48. Paice J, Penn R. Practices related to the use of implanted pumps for intraspinal drug delivery for pain: a survey. Presentation at American Pain Society 12th Annual Scientific Meeting; 1993: *A-38*.

49. Paice J, Buck M. Intraspinal devices for pain management. *Nurs Clin North Am*. 1993; 28(4):921–935.

50. Davidoff RA, Sears ED. The effects of Lioresal on synaptic activity in the isolated spinal cord. *Neurology*. 1974; 24:957–963.

51. Penn R, Kroin J. Intrathecal baclofen in the long-term management of severe spasticity. *Neurosurgery*. 1989; 4(2):325–332.

52. Wilson PR, Yaksh TL. Baclofen is antinociceptive in the spinal intrathecal space of animals. *Eur J Pharmacol*. 1978; 51(4): 323–330.

53. Yaksh TL, Reddy SVR. Studies in the primate on the analgesic effects associated with intrathecal actions of opiates, alpha-adrenergic agonists and baclofen. *Anesthesiology*. 1981; 54(6): 451–467.

54. Kroin JS, Penn RD, Beissinger RL, et al. Reduced spinal reflexes following intrathecal baclofen in the rabbit. *Exp Brain Res*. 1984; 54(1):191–194.

55. Borner U, Müller H, Zierski J, et al. CSF compatibility of antispastic agents. In: Müller H, Zierski J, Penn R D (eds). *Local-Spinal Therapy of Spasticity*. Berlin, Germany: Springer-Verlag; 1988: 81–84.

56. Penn RD, Kroin JS. Intrathecal baclofen alleviates spinal cord spasticity. *Lancet*. 1984; i(8385):1078.

57. Penn RD, Kroin JS. Long-term intrathecal baclofen infusion for treatment of spasticity. *J Neurosurg*. 1987; 66(2):181–185.

58. Delhaas E, Verhagen J. Pregnancy in a quadriplegic patient treated with continuous intrathecal baclofen infusion to manage her severe spasticity. Case report. *Paraplegia*. 1992; 30:527–528.

59. Atweh S, Kuhar M. Autoradiographic localization of opiate receptors in rat brain. I. Spinal cord and lower medulla. *Brain Res*. 1977; 124(1):53–67.

60. Yaksh TL, Rudy TA. Chronic catheterization of the spinal subarachnoid space. *Physiol Behav*. 1976; 17:1031–1036.

61. Yaksh T. Analgetic actions of intrathecal opiates in cats and primates. *Brain Res*. 1978; 153(1):205–210.

62. Coombs DW, Fratkin JD, Meier FA. Neuropathologic lesions and CSF morphine concentrations during chronic continuous intraspinal morphine infusion. A clinical and post-mortem study. *Pain* 1985; 22:337–351.

63. Moulin DE, Inturrisi CE, Foley KM. Cerebrospinal fluid pharmacokinetics of intrathecal morphine sulfate and D-Ala^5-D-Leu^5-enkephalin. *Ann Neurol*. 1986; 20(22):218–222.

64. Sabbe M, Grafe M, Mjanger E, et al. Spinal delivery of sufentanil, alfentanil, and morphine in dogs. *Anesthesiology.* 1994; 81(4): 899–920.

65. Butterworth J, Strichartz G. Molecular mechanisms of local anesthesia: a review. *Anesthesiology.* 1990; 72(4):711–734.

66. Cousins M, Bromage P. Epidural neural blockade. In: Cousins M, Bridenbaugh P (eds). *Neural Blockade in Clinical Anesthesia and Management of Pain.* Philadelphia, Pa: Lippincott; 1988: 253–360.

67. Berde C, Sethna N, Conrad L. Subarachnoid bupivicaine analgesia for seven months for a patient with a spinal cord tumor. *Anesthesiology.* 1990; 72(6):1094–1096.

68. DuPen S, Williams A. Management of patients receiving combined epidural morphine and bupivicaine for the treatment of cancer pain. *J Pain Symptom Manage.* 1992; 7(2):125–127.

69. DuPen S, Kharasch E, Williams A. Chronic epidural bupivicaine-opioid infusion in intractable cancer pain. *Pain.* 1992; 49(3): 293–300.

70. Nitescu P, Appelgren L, Lindner L. Epidural versus intrathecal morphine-bupivicaine: assessment of consecutive treatment in advanced cancer pain. *J Pain Symptom Manage.* 1990; 5(1):18–26.

71. Moulin D, Coyle N. Spinal opioid analgesics and local anesthetics in the management of chronic cancer pain. *J Pain Symptom Manage.* 1986; 1(2):79–86.

72. Sjoberg M, Appelgren L, Einarsson S, et al. Long-term intrathecal morphine and bupivicane in "refractory" cancer pain. I. Results from the first series of 52 patients. *Acta Anesthesiol Scand.* 1991; 35(1):30–43.

73. Raj P. Local anesthetic blockade. In Patt R (ed). *Cancer Pain.* Philadelphia, Pa: Lippincott; 1993: 334.

74. Akerman F, Arwestrom E, Post C. Local anesthetics potentiate spinal morphine antinociception. *Anesth Analg.* 1988; 67(10): 943–948.

75. Rigler M, Drasner K, Krejcie T, et al. Cauda equina syndrome after continuous spinal analgesia. *Anesth Analg.* 1991; 72:275–281.

76. Kroin JS, McCarthy RJ, Penn RD, et al. The effect of chronic subarachnoid bupivacaine infusion in dogs. *Anesthesiology.* 1987; 66(6):737–742.

77. Eisenach J, Rauck R, Buzzanell C, et al. Epidural clonidine analgesia for intractable cancer pain: phase I. *Anesthesiology.* 1989; 71(5):647–652.

78. Glynn C, Dawon D, Sanders R. A double-blind comparison between epidural morphine and epidural clonidine in patients with chronic non-cancer pain. *Pain.* 1988; 34(2):123–128.

79. Coombs D, Saunders R, Fratkin J, et al. Continuous intrathecal

hydromorphone and clonidine for intractable cancer pain. *J Neurosurg.* 1986; 64(6):890–894.

80. McCarthy RJ, Kroin JS, Lubenow TR, et al. Effect of intrathecal tizanidine on antinociception and blood pressure in the rat. *Pain.* 1990; 40(3):333–338.

81. Rosenthal B, Ho R. An electron microscopic study of somatostatin immunoreactive structures in lamina II of the rat spinal cord. *Brain Res Bull.* 1989; 22(2):439–451.

82. Randic M, Miletic V. Depressant actions of methionine-enkephalin and somatostatin in the cat dorsal horn neurones activated by noxious stimuli. *Brain Res.* 1978; 152(1):196–202.

83. Chrubasik J, Meynadier J, Blond S, et al. Somatostatin, a potent analgesic. *Lancet.* 1984; ii(8413):1208–1209.

84. Penn RD, Paice JA, Kroin JS. Octreotide: a potent new non-opiate analgesic for intrathecal infusion. *Pain.* 1992; 49(1):13–19.

85. Poli P, Sabbia E, Venturi L. Intrathecal octreotide for cancer pain: our experience. *7th World Congress on Pain Abstr.* 1993; 215:76–77.

86. Chapman V, Dickenson A. The combination of NMDA antagonism and morphine produces profound antinociception in the rat dorsal horn. *Brain Res.* 1992; 573(2):321–323.

87. Malinovsky J, Cozian A, Lepage J. Ketamine and midazolam neurotoxicity in the rabbit. *Anesthesiology.* 1991; 75(1):91–97.

88. Borgbjerg F, Svensson B, Frigast C, et al. Histopathology after repeated intrathecal injections of preservative-free ketamine in the rabbit: a light and electron microscopic examination. *Anesth Analg.* 1994; 79(1):105–111.

89. Wiesendanger M. Neurophysiological basis of spasticity. In Sindou M, Abbott R, Kerevel Y (eds): *Neurosurgery for Spasticity.* New York, NY: Springer-Verlag; 1991: 15–19.

90. Lance J. Pathophysiology of spasticity and clinical experience with baclofen. In: Feldman R, Young R, Koella W (eds). *Spasticity: Disordered Motor Control.* Chicago, Ill: Year Book Medical Publishers; 1980: 185–203.

91. McKeough D. *The coloring review of neuroscience.* Boston, Mass: Little, Brown and Company; 1982.

92. Little JW, Micklesen P, Umlauf R, Britell C. Lower extremity manifestations of spasticity in chronic spinal cord injury. *Am J Phys Med Rehabil.* 1989; 68(1):32–36.

93. Hattab JR. Review of European clinical trials with baclofen. In Feldman RG, Young RR, Kaella WP (eds). *Spasticity: Disordered Motor Control.* Miami. Fla: Symposia Specialists; 1980: 71–85.

94. Penn RD, Corcos DM. Spasticity and its management. In Youmans JR (ed). *Neurological Surgery.* Philadelphia, Pa: W. B. Saunders

Company; 1990: 4371-4385.

95. Knutsson E, Lindbloom U, Martensson A. Plasma and cerebrospinal fluid levels of baclofen (Lioresal) at optimal therapeutic responses in spastic paresis. *J Neurol Sci.* 1974; 23(3):473-484.

96. Costa E, Givdotti A. Molecular mechanisms in the receptor action of benzodiazepines. *Annu Rev Pharmacol Toxicol.* 1979; 19:531-54.

97. Ellis K, Bryant S. Excitation-contraction uncoupling in skeletal muscle by dantrolene sodium. *Naunyn Schmeidebergs Arh Pharmakol.* 1972; 274(1):107-109.

98. Ellis K, Carpenter J. Studies on the mechanisms of action of dantrolene sodium. A skeletal muscle relaxant. *Naunyn Schmeidebergs Arh Pharmakol.* 1972; 275:83-94.

99. Young J, Mayer R. Physiological alterations of motor units in hemiplegia. *J Neurosci.* 1982; 54:401-412.

100. Young RR, Delwaide PJ. Drug therapy: spasticity (first of two parts). *N Engl J Med.* 1981; 304(1):28-33.

101. Tremblay L, Bedard P. Effect of clonidine on motorneuron excitability in spinalized rats. *Neuropharmacology.* 1986; 25(1):41-46.

102. Donovan W, Carter R, Rossi C, et al. Clonidine effect on spasticity: a clinical trial. *Arch Phys Med Rehabil.* 1988; 69(3, Pt 1):193-194.

103. Weingarden S, Belen J. Clonidine transdermal system for treatment of spasticity in spinal cord injury. *Arch Phys Med Rehabil.* 1992; 73(9):876-877.

104. Knutsson E, Martenson A, Grossberg L. Antiparetic and antispastic effects induced by tizanidine in patients with spastic paresis. *J Neurol Sci.* 1982; 53(2):187-204.

105. Mathias C, Luckitt J, Desai P, et al. Pharmacodynamics and pharmacokinetics of the oral antispastic agent tizanidine in patients with spinal cord injury. *J Rehab Res Dev.* 1989; 26(4):9-16.

106. Dimitrijevic M, Dimitrijevic M, Illis L, et al. Spinal cord stimulation for the control of spasticity in patients with chronic spinal cord injury: I. Clinical observations. *Cent Nerv Syst Trauma.* 1986; 3(2):129-144.

107. Gottlieb GL, Myklebust BM, Stefoski D, et al. Evaluation of cervical stimulation for chronic treatment of spasticity. *Neurology.* 1985; 35(5):699-704.

108. Cooper I, Riklan M, Amin I, et al. Chronic cerebellar stimulation in cerebral palsy. *Neurology.* 1976; 26(8):744-753.

109. Fisher MA, Penn RD. Evidence for changes in segmental motorneuron pools by chronic cerebellar stimulation and its clinical significance. *J Neurol Neurosurg Psychiatry.* 1978; 41(7):630-635.

110. Penn RD. Chronic cerebellar stimulation for cerebral palsy: a review. *Neurosurgery.* 1982; 10(1):116-121.

111. Erickson DL, Blacklock JB, Michaelson M, et al. Control of

spasticity by implantable continuous flow morphine pump. *Neuro-surgery.* 1985; 15(2):215–217.

112. Chabal C, Jacobson L, Termon G. Intrathecal fentanyl alleviates spasticity in the presence of tolerance to intrathecal baclofen. *Anesthesiology.* 1992; 76(2):312–314.

113. Kasdon DL. Controversies in the surgical management of spasticity. *Clin Neurosurg* 1986; 35:523–529.

114. Penn RD, Savoy S, Corcos D, et al. Intrathecal baclofen for severe spinal spasticity: a double-blind crossover study. *N Engl J Med.* 1989; 320(23):1517–1521.

115. Loubser PG, Narayan RK, Sandin KJ, et al. Continuous infusion of intrathecal baclofen: long-term effects on spasticity in spinal cord injury. *Paraplegia.* 1991; 29(1):48–64.

116. Ochs G, Struppler A, Meyerson BA, et al. Intrathecal baclofen for long-term treatment of spasticity: a multi-centre study. *J Neurol Neurosurg Psychiatry.* 1989; 52(8):933–939.

117. Lazorthes Y, Sallerin-Caute B, Verdie JC, et al. Chronic intrathecal baclofen administration for control of severe spasticity. *J Neurosurg.* 1990; 72(3):393–402.

118. Müller H. Treatment of severe spasticity: results of a multicenter trial conducted in Germany involving the intrathecal infusion of baclofen by an implantable drug delivery system. *RBM.* 1991; 13:184–186.

119. Parke B, Penn RD, Savoy SM, et al. Functional outcome after delivery of intrathecal baclofen. *Arch Phys Med Rehabil.* 1989; 70(1):30–32.

120. Steers W, Meythaler J, Haworth C, et al. Effects of acute bolus and chronic continuous intrathecal baclofen on genitourinary dysfunction due to spinal cord pathology. *J Urol.* 1992; 148(6):1849–1855.

121. Frost F, Nanninga JB, Penn RD, et al. Intrathecal baclofen infusion: effect on bladder management programs in patients with myelopathy. *Am J Phys Med Rehabil.* 1989; 68(3):112–115.

122. Talalla A, Grundy D, Macdonnell R. The effect of intrathecal baclofen on the lower urinary tract in paraplegia. *Paraplegia.* 1990; 28:420–427.

123. Taira T, Tanikawa T, Kawamura H, Iseki H, Takakura K. Spinal intrathecal baclofen suppresses central pain after a stroke. *J Neurol Neurosurg Psychiatry* 1994; 57(3):381–382.

124. Kravitz HM, Corcos DM, Hanson G, Penn RD, Cartwright RD, Gianino J. Intrathecal baclofen effects on nocturnal leg muscle spasticity. *Am J Phys Med Rehabil.* 1992; 71(1):48–52.

125. Latash ML, Penn RD, Corcos DM, et al. Short-term effects of intrathecal baclofen in spasticity. *Exp Neurol.* 1989; 103(2):165–172.

126. Ashworth B. Preliminary trial of carisoprodol in multiple sclerosis. *Practitioner.* 1964; 192:540–542.
127. Penn RD, Kroin JS. Continuous intrathecal baclofen for severe spasticity. *Lancet.* 1985; ii(8447):125–127.
128. Savoy S, Gianino J. Intrathecal baclofen infusion: an innovative approach for controlling spinal spasticity. *Rehabil Nurs.* 1993; 18(2):105–113.
129. Penn R, Gianino J, York M. Intrathecal baclofen in motor disorders. *Mov Disord.* 1995; 10(6): In press.
130. Albright A, Barron W, Fasick M, et al. Continuous intrathecal baclofen infusion for spasticity of cerebral origin. *JAMA* 1993; 270(20):2475.
131. Albright LA, Cervi A, Singletary J. Intrathecal baclofen for spasticity in cerebral palsy. *JAMA* 1991; 265(11):1418–1422.
132. Rawlins P. Intrathecal baclofen for spasticity of cerebral palsy: project coordination and nursing care. *J Neurosci Nurs.* 1995; 27(3):157–163.
133. Penn R, Mangieri E. Stiff-man syndrome treated with intrathecal baclofen. *Neurology.* 1993; 43(11):2412.
134. Ford, Fahn: Letter to the editor. *Neurology.* 1994; 44(7):1367–8.
135. Narayan R, Loubser P, Jankovic J, et al. Intrathecal baclofen for intractable axial dystonia. *Neurology.* 1991; 41(7):1141–1142.
136. Mandac B, Hurvitz E, Nelson V. Hyperthermia associated with baclofen withdrawal and increased spasticity. *Arch Phys Med Rehabil.* 1993; 74(1):96–97.
137. Kofler M, Leis A. Prolonged seizure activity after baclofen withdrawal. *Neurology.* 1992; 42(3, Pt 1):697–698.
138. Terrence C, Fromm G. Complications of baclofen withdrawal. *Arch Neurol.* 1981; 38(9):588–589.
139. Gianino J. Intrathecal baclofen for spinal spasticity: implications for nursing practice. *J Neurosci Nurs.* 1993; 24(4):254–264.
140. Siegfried R, Jacobson L, Chabal C. Development of an acute withdrawal syndrome following the cessation of intrathecal baclofen in a patient with spasticity. *Anesthesiology.* 1992; 77:1048–1050.
141. Müller-Schwefe G, Penn RD. Physostigmine in the treatment of intrathecal baclofen overdose: report of three cases. *J Neurosurg.* 1989; 71:273–275.
142. Newton R. Physostigmine salicyate in the treatment of trycyclic antidepressant overdose. *JAMA.* 1975; 231(9):941–943.
143. Nilsson E. Physostigmine treatment in various drug-induced intoxications. *Ann Clin Res.* 1982; 14(4):165–172.
144. Giacobini E. Pharmacokinetics and pharmacodynamics of physostigmine after intravenous administration in beagle dogs. *Neuro-*

pharmacology. 1987; 26(7B):831–836.

145. Delhaas EM, Brouwers JRBJ. Intrathecal baclofen overdose: report of 7 events in 5 patients and review of the literature. *Int J Clin Pharmacol Ther Toxicol.* 1991; 29(7):274–280.

146. Saltuari L, Marosi MJ, Kofler M, et al. Status epilepticus complicating intrathecal baclofen overdose. *Lancet.* 1992; 339(8789): 373–374.

147. Penn RD, Kroin JS, Magolan JM. Intrathecal baclofen in the treatment of spinal spasticity. *Clin Neuropharmacol.* 1990; 13(2):400–401.

148. Kroin J, Bianchi G, Penn R. Intrathecal baclofen down-regulates $GABA_B$ receptors in the rat substantia gelatinosa. *J Neurosurg.* 1993; 79:544–549.

149. Erickson D, Lo J, Michaelson M. Control of intractable spasticity with intrathecal morphine sulfate. *Neurosurgery.* 1989; 24(2): 236–238.

150. Hennan R, Wainberg M, Guidice PD, et al. The effect of low dose intrathecal morphine sulfate on impaired micturition reflexes in human subjects with spinal cord lesions. *Anesthesiology.* 1988; 69:313–318.

151. Chabal C, Jacobson L, Schwid H. An objective comparison of intrathecal lidocaine versus fentanyl for the treatment of lower extremity spasticity. *Anesthesiology.* 1991; 74(4):643–646.

152. International Association for the study of Pain. 1979.

153. Jacox A, Carr D, Payne R, et al. *Management of Cancer Pain: Clinical Practice Guideline.* Vol 9. Rockville, Md: US Dept of Health and Human Services; 1994.

154. Fields H. *Pain.* New York, NY: McGraw-Hill Book Company; 1987.

155. Max MB, Inturrisi CE, Kaiko RF, et al. Epidural and intrathecal opiates: cerebrospinal fluid plasma profiles in patients with chronic cancer pain. *Clin Pharmacol Ther.* 1985; 38(6):631–641.

156. Auld A, Maki-Jokela A, Murdoch D. Intraspinal narcotic analgesia in the treatment of chronic pain. *Spine.* 1985; 10(8):777–781.

157. Brazenor G. Long term intrathecal administration of morphine: a comparison of bolus injection via reservoir with continuous infusion by implanted pump. *Neurosurgery.* 1987; 21(4):484–491.

158. Coombs DW, Maurer LH, Saunders RL, et al. Outcomes and complications of continuous intraspinal narcotic analgesia for cancer pain control. *J Clin Oncol.* 1984; 2(12):1414–1420.

159. Coombs DW, Saunders RL, Gaylor MS, et al. Epidural narcotic infusion reservoir: implantation technique and efficacy. *Anesthesiology.* 1982; 56(6):469–473.

160. Coombs DW, Saunders RL, Gaylor MS. Relief of continuous

chronic pain by intraspinal narcotics via an implanted reservoir. *JAMA*. 1983; 250(17):2336.

161. Follett K, Hitchon P, Piper J, et al. Response of intractable pain to continuous intrathecal morphine: a retrospective study. *Pain*. 1992; 49(1):21–25.

162. Hassenbusch S, Pillay P, Magdinec M, et al. Constant infusion of morphine for intractable cancer pain using an implanted pump. *J Neurosurg*. 1990; 73(3):405–409.

163. Krames ES, Gershow J, Glassberg A, et al. Continuous infusion of spinally administered narcotics for the relief of pain due to malignant disorders. *Cancer*. 1985; 56(3):696–702.

164. Onofrio BM, Yaksh TL, Arnold PG. Continuous low-dose intrathecal morphine administration in the treatment of chronic pain of malignant origin. *Mayo Clin Proc*. 1981; 56(8):516–520.

165. Penn RD, Paice JA. Chronic intrathecal morphine for intractable pain. *J Neurosurg*. 1987; 67(2):182–186.

166. Penn RD, Paice JA, Gottshalk W, et al. Cancer pain relief using chronic morphine infusion: early experience with a programmable implanted drug pump. *J Neurosurg*. 1984; 61(2):302–306

167. Shetter AG. Administration of intraspinal morphine sulfate for the treatment of intractable cancer pain. *Neurosurgery*. 1986; 18(6):740–747.

168. Waterman N, Hughes S, Foster W. Control of cancer pain by epidural infusion of morphine. *Surgery*. 1991; 110(4):612–616.

169. Maniker A, Krieger A, Adler R, et al. Epidural trial in implantation of intrathecal morphine infusion pumps. *NJ Med*. 1991; 88(11): 797–801.

170. Turner J, Deyo R, Loeser J, et al. The importance of placebo effects in pain treatment and research. *JAMA*. 1994; 271(20):1609–1614.

171. Paice J, Penn R, Shott S. Intrathecal morphine for chronic pain: a retrospective, multicenter study. Accepted for publication. *J Pain Manage*.

172. Nordberg G. Pharmacokinetic aspects of spinal morphine analgesia. *Acta Anaesthesiol Scand*. 1984; 79(28):7–32.

173. Yaksh T, Onofrio B. Retrospective consideration of the doses of morphine given intrathecally by chronic infusion in 163 patients by 19 physicians. *Pain*. 1987; 31(2)211–223.

174. VanDongen R, Crul B, DeBock M. Long-term intrathecal infusion of morphine and morphine/bupivicaine mixtures in the treatment of cancer pain: a retrospective analysis of 51 cases. *Pain*. 1993; 55(1):119–123.

175. Schultheiss R, Schramm J, Neidhardt J. Dose changes in long- and medium-term intrathecal morphine therapy of cancer pain. *Neurosurgery*. 1992; 31(4):664–670.

176. Caputi C, Busca G, Fogliardi A, et al. Evaluation of tolerance in long-term treatment of cancer pain with epidural morphine. *Int J Clin Pharmacol Ther Toxicicol.* 1983; 21(11):587–590.

177. Paice J, Penn R, Ryan W. Altered sexual function and decreased testosterone in patients receiving intraspinal opioids. *J Pain Symptom Manage.* 1994; 9(2):126–131.

178. Penn RD. Intrathecal baclofen for spasticity of spinal origin: seven years of experience. *J Neurosurg.* 1992; 77(2):236–240.

179. Penn RD, York MM, Paice JA. Catheter systems for intrathecol drug delivery. *J Neurosurg.* 1995; 83(2):215–217.

180. Rosenson A, Ali A, Fordham E, et al. Indium-111 DPTA flow study to evaluate surgically implanted drug delivery system. *Clin Nucl Med.* 1990; 15(3):154–156.

181. Medtronic: *Overview of Therapy, Benefits and Costs. Lioresal Intrathecal SynchroMed Infusion Pump.* 1992.

182. Bedder M, Burchiel K, Larson A. Cost analysis of two implantable narcotic delivery systems. *J Pain Symptom Manage.* 1991; 6(6):368–373.

Appendix 1. Baclofen Patient Teaching Booklet

For many people spasticity can be so devastating that it creates pain, limits sleep, makes it difficult to transfer, and even makes it hard or impossible to perform simple everyday tasks. Baclofen, more commonly known as Lioresal, is an antispastic agent that can be taken in the pill form to help decrease spasticity. Unfortunately, oral baclofen may not be effective in reducing spasticity, and high doses may produce intolerable side effects.

Since 1984 we have been testing the effectiveness of baclofen in a liquid form that is given directly into the spine. The results have been dramatic, with a decrease in spasms and rigidity.

A simple operation using local anesthesia is performed to insert a catheter in the spine and to implant a pump in the abdomen. The pump can deliver medication through a catheter directly into the spine, where it is needed to relieve intractable spasticity.

Suitable Candidates

A candidate for this therapy must have intractable spasticity (i.e., spasticity that has not responded to oral medications such as Lioresal, Dantrium, or Valium).

You cannot use this therapy if you have an allergy to oral baclofen (Lioresal). Caution is needed if you plan on becoming pregnant or have another implanted programmable device (e.g., cardiac pacemaker).

Liquid Baclofen

Baclofen, also known as Lioresal, is an antispastic medication that relieves spasticity and the pain associated with it. Baclofen works directly on the spinal cord to reduce the aggravation of the nerve cells by stopping the signals that irritate the muscle. The muscles are then able to relax.

When taking baclofen in the pill form, it is absorbed into the bloodstream and distributed throughout the body. Because it is distributed in different parts of the body, this may sometimes cause side effects (e.g., drowsiness, dizziness, or nausea). Baclofen in the *liquid* form can be given directly into the intrathecal space of the spinal cord, making it much more powerful than in the pill form. And there are no side effects since the liquid baclofen goes directly to the spinal fluid and not into the bloodstream.

This new form of baclofen delivered into the intrathecal space is a major breakthrough for those who are not being helped by oral antispasmodics or who have unwanted side effects while taking them.

It is important to understand that while this form of baclofen may reduce spasticity, it is not a cure for a disease, nor will it provide strength.

What Does Intrathecal Mean?

The term "intrathecal" refers to the space along the spinal cord into which baclofen is delivered. The intrathecal space is where the cerebrospinal fluid (CSF) flows. The CSF is a clear fluid that is produced within the ventricles of the brain. The CSF circulates around the brain and spinal cord, acting as a shock absorber to protect these delicate structures. Baclofen in its liquid form will be delivered into this space in the lower back. The liquid baclofen will mix with the fluid from the spine (CSF). This will be absorbed in the spinal tissues, where it will work directly in the spine to reduce the spasticity.

How Is Baclofen Delivered into the Intrathecal Space?

Baclofen is delivered continuously along the spinal cord by an implantable drug pump system. The system consists of two parts: a pump and a catheter.

Pump and Catheter

The pump is a round, metal disk which weighs about 6 oz and measures about 1 inch thick and 3 inches in diameter. The pump is battery operated and is constructed with a reservoir that holds a specific volume of the liquid baclofen. Battery life is dose dependent and ranges from 3 to 5 years. When the battery is low, the pump needs to be replaced.

Safety mechanisms such as an alarm system and bacterioretentive filter are built into the pump. The separate alarms will sound when the battery is low and when the reservoir is empty of the medication. The bacterioretentive filter is essential because it *eliminates* the possibility of contaminants (e.g., bacteria) from being delivered with the medication into the spine.

The pump is surgically placed into the lower abdomen. It may protrude from the abdomen. The pump should not interfere with movement or cause any discomfort. The pump is connected to a catheter that is tunneled around the side of the body, leading to the lumbar, or lower, part of the spine. The entire pump and catheter remain sterile, just beneath the surface of the skin.

Baclofen Dose Adjustments

A portable computer programs the pump to deliver medications at varying rates. Through a high-frequency radio wave, a programming wand reads and resets the pump status when programmed. This is known as "telemetry." The dose of baclofen is adjusted by holding the programming wand near the skin over the pump. It allows the doctor or nurse to precisely program doses that facilitate optimal functioning (i.e., the pump can be programmed to deliver more baclofen at times when spasticity is greater). Also, these radio signals indicate how accurately the pump is operating.

What Happens When the Pump Runs Out of Baclofen?

The pump needs to be refilled when it runs out of baclofen. Refilling the pump is a simple procedure performed in the doctor's office. In the center of the pump is a raised portion that helps the doctor or nurse find the filling port. In the middle of the filling port is a self-sealing, rubber septum. A needle is inserted through the skin, then through the septum to refill the pump with baclofen. Frequency of refills is determined by the amount of baclofen needed to control spasticity for each individual, averaging every 4 to 12 weeks.

The Screening Phase

An examination in our office will be needed to assess spasticity to see if you are a candidate. The next screening phase takes place in the hospital. Videotaping and tests will be done before and after the trial dose of intrathecal baclofen. The trial dose is given through the spinal cord by a procedure called a lumbar puncture or spinal tap. If the trial dose of intrathecal baclofen reduces spasticity, you will have the option to proceed with the surgery for the implantation of a pump. If the trial dose does not reduce spasticity, a higher dose of intrathecal baclofen may be tried.

Surgical Phase

Placing the drug pump superficially into the abdomen and tunneling the catheter from the pump into the spine is a minor surgical procedure lasting approximately 2 hours. This procedure can be performed with local anesthesia and supplemental intravenous medication; however, general anesthesia may be warranted. Two surgical incisions are needed: one incision in the abdomen for the pump, and one incision in the back for insertion of the catheter into the spine. There is no reason to avoid lying on the abdomen after the incision has healed and tenderness over the pump has diminished. There are no activity restrictions. The estimated length of the hospital stay is approximately 4 to 5 days.

Postoperatively doses of oral antispastic medications will be *gradually* discontinued. Doses of intrathecal baclofen will be programmed to meet individual needs. Discharge instructions will be provided regarding follow-up evaluation, refills, wound healing, and emergency procedures.

Advantages of Intrathecal Baclofen

There are several advantages of controlling spasticity with intrathecal baclofen. The greatest advantage is that the amount of baclofen can be precisely adjusted according to the individual's needs. Because *some* spasticity may enhance function and ambulation, flexibility with dosage adjusting is important. Also, baclofen is delivered directly into the lumbar spine, acting specifically where it is needed to reduce spasticity. The most common side effect reported with oral antispastic medications is drowsiness. This is rare when baclofen is administered intrathecally. The drug pump enables a constant level of baclofen to be maintained at the spinal level. The surgical procedure is nondestructive, preserving all vital links in the motor control. Lastly, the delivery system (pump and catheter) is not permanent, permitting future options for control of spasticity to be explored.

Overall View

Initial Office Visit for Assessment

Day 1: Testing with intrathecal baclofen

- Videotaping (before and after baclofen injection) may be necessary
- Testing at the motor lab (before and after baclofen injection) may be necessary
- Lumbar puncture (spinal tap) to administer liquid baclofen
- Continuous monitoring of heart rate and respirations
- Frequent evaluation of reflexes and spasms
- Assessment of effects from baclofen*

---

*If the baclofen has not significantly reduced spasticity, another trial of baclofen at a higher dose may be needed. If the trial of baclofen *has* significantly reduced spasticity, surgery will be scheduled for the next day.

Day 2: Surgery

- Performed under local anesthesia and intravenous sedatives to promote relaxation
- Lasts approximately 2 hours

Days 3–5: Postoperative period

- Resume previous diet and activities
- Frequent evaluation of spasticity
- Intrathecal baclofen dosage adjustments as necessary
- Decreasing oral baclofen (Lioresal)
- Daily checks of abdominal and back incisions

Discharge

- Approximately 2 to 3 days after surgery
- Written discharge instructions will be provided and reviewed
- Pump ID card will be issued

Follow-up

- Return to office 7 to 10 days after surgery for removal of sutures and evaluation of spasticity and pump's performance
- Return to office every 4 to 12 weeks for refill and dose adjustment

If you have any questions or concerns, please feel free to contact us.

(Name)   (Name)

Appendix 2.

Intrathecal Baclofen and Morphine: Policy and Procedure
Rush Presbyterian St. Luke's Medical Center
Chicago, Ill

SECTION: Medications

SUBJECT: *INTRATHECAL MEDICATION*
ADMINISTRATION VIA IMPLANTABLE
PUMP

INFORMATION:

1. Infusaid or Medtronic programmable pumps are used for the administration of intrathecal medications, which can be useful in the treatment of intractable pain or spasticity.

2. Temperature rise can increase rate of infusion when using Infusaid device.

3. Supplemental pain medicationss are allowed for patients who have undergone pump insertion.

4. Oral baclofen is decreased slowly to prevent possible seizures or hallucinations.

5. Pain scale: 0 = no pain;
   10 = worst pain imaginable

6. Scale for spasticity (Ashworth scale);
   1 = no ↑in tone;
   5 = extremely rigid
   Spasms (spasm scale) 0 = none;
   4 = > 10 spasms per hour

POLICY:

1. Preoperative pain assessment is made on each patient before insertion for implanted pump using 0–10 pain scale. Preoperative assessment of spasticity is made by the nurse clinicians in neurosurgery.

2. Patient is monitored for the first 24 hours with an apnea monitor or pulse oximetry.

   2.1. A cardiac monitor is used if an apnea monitor or pulse oximetry is unavailable.

3. Medication concentration is ordered and refilled only by physician or nurse clinicians associated with the project.

4. An assessment of pump site is documented on the appropriate patient care record every shift.

RESPONSIBILITY   PROCEDURE

RN

1. Make preoperative pain assessment on the patient using 0–10 pain scale.

Physician

2. Insert medication and pump in the OR.

RN

3. Apply apnea monitor/pulse oximetry to patient as ordered for initial 24-hour period or as ordered per physician.

Baclofen (spasticity)

3.1. Assess patient for episodes of decreased respirations, drowsiness, slurred speech, change in mentation, or other neurological changes.

3.2. Administer physostigmine as ordered.

3.3 Notify physician if any of the above symptoms occur.

Opiates (pain)

3.1. Assess patient for episodes of somnolence, respiratory depression.

3.2. Administer Narcan (naloxone) as ordered.

3.3. Notify physician if respiratory depression occurs.

4. Record vital signs and subjective pain level using the 0–10 pain scale post operatively every 4 hours for the first 8 hours, then at least every shift until patient is discharged.

5. Monitor intake & output.

   5.1. Report any episodes of urinary retention.

6. Report any episodes of pruritus.

7. Administer supplemental pain medication as ordered.

8. Assess site of incisions and pump site for signs and symptoms of infection every shift.

   8.1. Document assessment on appropriate care record.

9. Instruct patient to:

   9.1. Avoid extended periods of heat such as long baths and heating pads.

   9.2. Notify physician for any episodes of elevated temperature (101.5°C orally).

   9.3. Avoid any rough physical activity.

   9.4. Notify physician or nurse associate prior to plane travel.

10. Give pump care manual and temporary ID card to patient prior to discharge.

Appendix 3.
Resources for
Spasticity

Appendix 3.1. Patient Resources: Spasticity

National Multiple Sclerosis Society
  600 S. Federal, Suite 204
  Chicago,IL 60605
  (312) 922-8000

National Rehabilitation Association
  633 S. Washington Street
  Alexandria, VA 22314

National Spinal Cord Injury Association
  600 West Cummings Park, Suite 2000
  Woburn, MA 01801
  1-800-962-9629

Paralyzed Veterans of America
  801 18th Street NW
  Washington,DC 20006
  (202) USA-1300

Athletics:

National Handicapped Sports and Recreation Association
  4405 East West Highway, Suite 603
  Bethesda, MA 20814
  (301) 652-7505

National Wheelchair Athletic Association
  3617 Betty Drive, Suite S
  Colorado Springs, CO 80917
  (303) 597-8330

Appendix 3.2. Professional Resources: Spasticity

American Association of Spinal Cord Injury Nurses
75-20 Astoria Boulevard
Jackson Heights, NY 11370-1178

American Society for Handicapped Physicians
105 Morris Drive
Bastrop,LA 71220
(318) 281-4436

**Appendix 3.3. Patient Resources: Travel Assistance
for the Disabled**

Access/Abilities
P.O. Box 458
Mill Valley, CA 94942
(415) 388-3250

Helping Hand Tours
1314 Pennsylvania Ave. SE
Washington, DC 20003
(202) 546-9496

Mobility Tours
26 Court Street
Brooklyn, NY 11242
(718) 858-6021

Society for the Advancement of Travel for the Handicapped
26 Court Street
Brooklyn, NY 11242
(718) 858-5483

Travel Helpers, Ltd.
160 Duncan Mill Road
Don Mills, Ontario, Canada M3125
(416) 443-0583

Wheels on Tour, Inc.
20202 Cobasset Street, Suite 10
Canoga Park, CA 91306
(818) 882-0441

Appendix 4.
Resources for Pain

Appendix 4.1. Patient Resources: Pain

American Cancer Society, Inc.
  1599 Clifton Road, N.E.
  Atlanta, GA 30329-4251
  1-800-ACS-2345
  (Check the phone book for your local unit.)

American Chronic Pain Association
  P.O. Box 850
  Rocklin, CA 95677
  (916) 632-0922
  FAX: (916) 632-3208

American Self-Help Clearinghouse
  (201) 642-7101
  (Can help find support groups in your state specific to your problem.)

National Cancer Institute
  Office of Cancer Communications
  Building 31, Room 10A24
  Bethesda, MD 20892
  1-800-4-CANCER

National Chronic Pain Outreach Association
  7979 Old Georgetown Road, Suite 100
  Bethesda, MD 20814-2429
  (301) 652-4948

National Coalition for Cancer Survivorship
  1010 Wayne Avenue, 5th Floor
  Silver Spring, MD 20910
  (301) 650-8868

Other Sources of Information (Books):

Coles J. *Pain Relief: How to Say No to Acute, Chronic & Cancer Pain!* New York, NY: Mastermedia Ltd; 1993. (800) 334-8232.

Sridhar V. *Pain: A Four-Letter Word You Can Live With.* Vasudevan, Md: Montgomery Media, Inc.; 1993. (414) 223-4266.

Matthews ML. *Pain, The Challenge and the Gift.* Marti Lynn Matthews. Stillpoint Publishing; 1991. (800) 847-4014.

Stacy CB, Kaplan AS, Williams G Jr. *The Fight Against Pain.* Consumer Reports Books; 1992.

Long SS, Patt RB. *You Don't Have to Suffer.* New York, NY: Oxford University Press; 1994. (713) 792-6911.

Appendix 4.2. Professional Resources: Pain

American Pain Society
5700 Old Orchard Road
Skokie, IL 60077
(708) 966-5595

American Society of Pain Management Nurses
Bristol St., Suite 110
Costa Mesa, CA 92626
(714) 545-1305

International Association for the Study of Pain
909 NE 43rd Street, Suite 306
Seattle, WA 98105
(206) 547-6409

Appendix 5.
Research
Organizations

American Association for the Advancement of Science
  Project for the Handicapped in Science
  1515 Massachusetts Ave. NW
  Washington, DC 20005
  (202) 467-4400

American Paralysis Association
  99 Morris Avenue
  Springfield, NJ 07081
  (800) 225-0292

National Committee for Research in
  Neurological and Communicative Disorders
  3050 K Street NW, Suite 310
  Washington, DC 20007
  (202) 293-5453

National Institute of Neurological and
  Communicative Disorders and Stroke
  National Institute of Health
  Office of Scientific Health Reports
  Building 31, Room 8A-06
  9000 Rockville Pike
  Bethesda, MD 20892

National Multiple Sclerosis Society
  600 S. Federal
  Chicago, IL 60605

National Spinal Cord Injury Association
  Director of Research
  600 West Cummings Park, Suite 2000
  Woburn, MA 01801
  (800) 962-9629

Paralyzed Veterans of America
  Spinal Cord Research Foundation
  National Research Director
  801 18th Street NW
  Washington, DC 20006
  (202) 872-1300

Society for Neuroscience
  Executive Secretary
  11 DuPont Circle NW
  Suite 500
  Washington, DC 20036
  (202) 462-6688

Appendix 6.
Electronic Support
Groups

DIRLINE
  Office of Inquiries and Publications
  Management
  National Library of Medicine
  8600 Rockville Pike
  Bethesda, MD 20894
  (301) 496-6308 or (800) 272-4787

E.T. Net Coordinator
  Educational Technology Branch
  Lister Hill National Center for Biomedical Communications
  National Library of Medicine
  8600 Rockville Pike
  Bethesda, MD 20894
  (301) 496-0508

HelpNet for the Impaired, Inc.
  23146 Lorain Road,Suite 313
  North Olmsted, OH 44070
  (216) 356-1328 (voice)
  (216) 356-1431/1772/1872/1961
  (dataline)

Internet
  NSF Network Service Center
  BBN (Bolt Beranek and Newman, Inc.)
  10 Moulton Street
  Cambridge, MA 0218
  (617) 873-3400
  E-mail: nnsc@nnsc.nst.net

American Self-Help Clearinghouse
(for help in locating or developing a member-run self-help group)
In New Jersey: (201) 625-7101 (voice)
Elsewhere: (800) 367-6274 (voice)
(TDD Line (201) 625-9053)